STUDENT WORKBOOK TO

INTRODUCTION TO MEDICAL TERMINOLOGY

Second Edition

Ann Ehrlich
Carol L. Schroeder

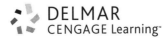
DELMAR
CENGAGE Learning™

Australia • Brazil • Japan • Korea • Mexico • Singapore • Spain • United Kingdom • United States

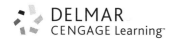
DELMAR
CENGAGE Learning™

Student Workbook to Accompany
Introduction to Medical Terminology
Second Edition
by Ann Ehrlich and Carol L. Schroeder

Vice President, Career and Professional Editorial: Dave Garza

Director of Learning Solutions: Matthew Kane

Acquisitions Editor: Matthew Seeley

Managing Editor: Marah Bellegarde

Senior Product Manager: Debra Myette-Flis

Editorial Assistant: Megan Tarquinio

Vice President, Career and Professional Marketing: Jennifer McAvey

Senior Marketing Manager: Michele McTighe

Production Director: Carolyn S. Miller

Content Project Manager: Thomas Heffernan

Senior Art Director: Jack Pendleton

Technology Project Manager: Benjamin Knapp

Production Technology Analyst: Tom Stover

For product information and technology assistance, contact us at
Professional & Career Group Customer Support, 1-800-648-7450

For permission to use material from this text or product, submit all requests online at **cengage.com/permissions.**
Further permissions questions can be e-mailed to **permissionrequest@cengage.com.**

Library of Congress Control Number: 2008926571

ISBN 13: 978-1-4180-3018-6
ISBN 10: 1-4180-3018-X

Delmar Cengage Learning
5 Maxwell Drive
Clifton Park, NY 12065-2919
USA

Cengage Learning products are represented in Canada by Nelson Education, Ltd.

For your lifelong learning solutions, visit **delmar.cengage.com**
Visit our corporate web site at **cengage.com.**

NOTICE TO THE READER

Publisher does not warrant or guarantee any of the products described herein or perform any independent analysis in connection with any of the product information contained herein. Publisher does not assume, and expressly disclaims, any obligation to obtain and include information other than that provided to it by the manufacturer. The reader is expressly warned to consider and adopt all safety precautions that might be indicated by the activities described herein and to avoid all potential hazards. By following the instructions contained herein, the reader willingly assumes all risks in connection with such instructions. The publisher makes no representations or warranties of any kind, including but not limited to, the warranties of fitness for particular purpose or merchantability, nor are any such representations implied with respect to the material set forth herein, and the publisher takes no responsibility with respect to such material. The publisher shall not be liable for any special, consequential, or exemplary damages resulting, in whole or part, from the readers' use of, or reliance upon, this material.

Printed in the United States of America
1 2 3 4 5 6 7 12 11 10 09 08

CONTENTS

TO THE STUDENT

Welcome to the *Student Workbook to Accompany Introduction to Medical Terminology*, Second Edition. This workbook contains many features to make your mastery of medical terminology easier, and it is to your benefit to take advantage of them.

CHAPTER ORGANIZATION

Flash Cards

The activity card pages at the back of this workbook are designed to be removed and used as flash cards. Flash cards are a great study aid, and early in your course you'll want to follow the instructions for removing these pages, separating the cards, and using them in a variety of fun study activities.

Chapter Features

There is a chapter in this workbook to accompany each chapter in your textbook. Each workbook chapter contains 100 Learning Exercises. To make these activities more interesting and challenging, they are in a variety of formats. With each question there is space for you to write your answer in the workbook. After you complete the exercises, follow your teacher's instructions for handing in your work and having it corrected. When these pages are returned to you, save them in your notebook for use as an additional review resource.

Writing the answer to each question, rather than just circling a letter, reinforces the material you are learning. Many questions include a variety of answer choices and you'll be pleasantly surprised at how quickly you can complete the exercises!

Word Part Review

There is a Word Part Review section to be completed after you have studied Chapters 1 and 2. This short section provides additional practice in working with word parts, plus a test to evaluate how well you've mastered their use.

Because most medical terms are based on word parts, mastery of these component's is very important before you begin your study of the body systems. If you have trouble here, this is the time to ask for help!

Comprehensive Review

At the end of your workbook there is a Comprehensive Medical Terminology Review section. This contains Study Tips, Review Questions, and a Simulated Final Test, all of which are designed to help you prepare for the final examination. You'll find this section very helpful when you use it on your own or in conjunction with class review sessions.

Good Luck!

It is our hope that your study of medical terminology will be interesting and rewarding. We also hope that the *Introduction to Medical Terminology* text and workbook help you find a career in health care that will bring you professional success and satisfaction.

Ann Ehrlich
Carol L. Schroeder

CHAPTER 1

Introduction to Medical Terminology

Learning Exercises

Class _____   Name _____

Matching Word Parts 1

Write the correct answer in the middle column.

Definition	Correct Answer	Possible Answers
1.1. bad, difficult, painful	_____	-algia
1.2. excessive, increased	_____	dys-
1.3. enlargement	_____	-ectomy
1.4. pain, suffering	_____	-megaly
1.5. surgical removal	_____	hyper-

Matching Word Parts 2

Write the correct answer in the middle column.

Definition	Correct Answer	Possible Answers
1.6. abnormal condition or disease	_____	hypo-
1.7. abnormal softening	_____	-itis
1.8. deficient, decreased	_____	-malacia
1.9. inflammation	_____	-necrosis
1.10. tissue death	_____	-osis

Matching Word Parts 3
Write the correct answer in the middle column.

Definition	Correct Answer	Possible Answers
1.11. bleeding, bursting forth	_____	-ostomy
1.12. creation of an artificial opening to the body surface	_____	-otomy
1.13. surgical incision	_____	-plasty
1.14. surgical repair	_____	-rrhage
1.15. surgical suturing	_____	-rrhaphy

Matching Word Parts 4
Write the correct answer in the middle column.

Definition	Correct Answer	Possible Answers
1.16. visual examination	_____	-rrhea
1.17. rupture	_____	-rrhexis
1.18. abnormal narrowing	_____	-sclerosis
1.19. abnormal hardening	_____	-scopy
1.20. flow or discharge	_____	-stenosis

Definitions
Select the correct answer and write it on the line provided.

1.21.   The term _____ describes any pathologic change or disease in the spinal cord.

   myelopathy   myopathy   pyelitis   pyrosis

1.22.   The medical term for higher than normal blood pressure is _____ .

   hepatomegaly   hypertension   hypotension   supination

1.23.   The term _____ means pertaining to birth.

   natal   perinatal   postnatal   prenatal

1.24.   Pain is classified as a _____ .

   diagnosis   sign   symptom   syndrome

1.25.   In the term myopathy, the suffix -pathy means _____ _____ .

   abnormal condition   disease   inflammation   swelling

Matching Terms and Definitions 1
Write the correct answer in the middle column.

Definition	Correct Answer	Possible Answers
1.26. white blood cell	_____	acute
1.27. prediction of the outcome of a disease	_____	edema
1.28. swelling caused by excess fluid in the body tissues	_____	leukocyte
1.29. sudden onset	_____	prognosis
1.30. turning the palm of the hand upward	_____	supination

Matching Terms and Definitions 2

Write the correct answer in the middle column.

Definition	Correct Answer	Possible Answers
1.31. examination procedure	_____	laceration
1.32. male gland	_____	lesion
1.33. pathologic tissue change	_____	palpitation
1.34. pounding heart	_____	palpation
1.35. torn, ragged wound, or an accidental cut wound	_____	prostate

Which Word?

Select the correct answer and write it on the line provided.

1.36. The medical term _____ describes an inflammation of the stomach.

gastritis   gastrosis

1.37. The formation of pus is called _____ .

supination   suppuration

1.38. The term meaning wound or injury is _____ .

trauma   triage

1.39. The term _____ means pertaining to a virus.

viral   virile

1.40. An _____ is the surgical removal of the appendix.

appendectomy   appendicitis

Spelling Counts

Find the misspelled word in each sentence. Then write that word, spelled correctly, on the line provided.

1.41. A disease named for the person who discovered it is known as an enaponym. _____

1.42. A localized response to injury or tissue destruction is called inflimmation. _____

1.43. A fisure of the skin is a groove or crack-like sore of the skin. _____

1.44. The medical term meaning the inflammation of a nerve or nerves is neuroitis. _____

1.45. The medical term meaning inflammation of the tonsils is tonsilitis. _____

Matching Terms

Write the correct answer in the middle column.

Definition	Correct Answer	Possible Answers
1.46. abnormal condition or disease of the stomach	_____	syndrome
1.47. a set of signs and symptoms	_____	gastralgia
1.48. rupture of a muscle	_____	gastrosis
1.49. stomach pain	_____	pyoderma
1.50. any acute pus-forming bacterial skin infection	_____	myorrhexis

Term Selection

Select the correct answer and write it on the line provided.

1.51. The abnormal hardening of the walls of an artery or arteries is called _____ .

   arteriosclerosis   arteriostenosis   arthrostenosis   atherosclerosis

1.52. A fever is considered to be a _____ .

   prognosis   sign   symptom   syndrome

1.53. An inflammation of the stomach and small intestine is known as _____ .

   gastralgia   gastroenteritis   gastritis   gastrosis

1.54. The term meaning pain in a joint or joints is _____ .

   arthralgia   arthritis   arthrocentesis   atherosclerosis

1.55. A _____ is a physician who specializes in diagnosing and treating diseases and disorders of the skin.

   dermatologist   dermatology   neurologist   neurology

Sentence Completion

Write the correct term on the line provided.

1.56. Lower than normal blood pressure is called _____ .

1.57. The process of recording a radiographic study of the blood vessels after the injection of a contrast medium is known as _____ .

1.58. The term meaning above or outside the ribs is _____ .

1.59. A/An _____ diagnosis is also known as a rule out.

1.60. A/An _____ is an abnormal passage, usually between two internal organs, or leading from an organ to the surface of the body.

True/False

If the statement is true, write **True** on the line. If the statement is false, write **False** on the line.

1.61. _____ An erythrocyte is commonly known as a red blood cell.

1.62. _____ Arteriomalacia is abnormal hardening of blood vessels of the walls of an artery or arteries.

1.63. _____ A colostomy is the surgical creation of an opening between the colon and the body surface.

1.64. _____ Malaise is often the first symptom of inflammation.

1.65. _____ An infection is the invasion of the body by a disease producing organism.

Word Surgery

Divide each term into its component word parts. Write these word parts, in sequence, on the lines provided. When necessary, use a slash (/) to indicate a combining vowel. (You may not need all of the lines provided.)

1.66. **Otorhinolaryngology** is the study of the ears, nose, and throat.

   _____   _____   _____   _____

1.67. The term **mycosis** means any abnormal condition or disease caused by a fungus.

   _____   _____   _____   _____

1.68. **Poliomyelitis** is a viral infection of the gray matter of the spinal cord.

_____ _____ _____ _____

1.68. **Neonatology** is the study of disorders of the newborn.

_____ _____ _____ _____

1.70. The term **endarterial** means pertaining to the interior or lining of an artery.

_____ _____ _____ _____

Clinical Conditions

Write the correct answer on the line provided.

1.71. Miguel required a/an _____ injection. This term means that the medication was placed directly within the muscle.

1.72. Mrs. Tillson underwent _____ to remove excess fluid from her abdomen.

1.73. The term **laser** is a/an _____ . This means that it is a word formed from the initial letter of the major parts of a compound term.

1.74. In the accident Felipe Valladares broke several bones in his fingers. The medical term for these injuries is fractured _____ .

1.75. In case of a major disaster Cheng Lee, who is a trained paramedic, helps to perform

_____ . This is the screening of patients to determine their relative priority of need and the proper place of treatment.

1.76. Ginaís physician ordered laboratory tests that would enable him to establish a differential

_____ to identify the cause of her signs and symptoms.

1.77. Jennifer plans to go to graduate school so she can specialize in _____ . This specialty is concerned with the study of all aspects of diseases.

1.78. John Randolphís cancer went into _____ . Although this is not a cure, his symptoms disappeared and he felt much better.

1.79. Mr. Jankowski describes that uncomfortable feeling as heartburn. The medical term for this condition

is _____ .

1.80. Phyllis was having a great fun traveling until she ate some contaminated food and developed

_____ . She felt miserable and needed to stay in her hotel because of the frequent flow of loose or watery stools.

Which Is the Correct Medical Term?

Select the correct answer and write it on the line provided.

1.81. The term _____ describes the surgical repair of a nerve.

neuralgia   neuritis   neurology   neuroplasty

1.82. The term _____ means loss of a large amount of blood in a short time.

diarrhea   hemorrhage   hepatorrhagia   otorrhagia

1.83. The term _____ means the tissue death of an artery or arteries.

arteriomalacia   arterionecrosis   arteriosclerosis   arteriostenosis

1.84. The term _____ means between, but not within, the parts of a tissue.

interstitial   intrastitial   intermuscular   intramuscular

1.85. The term _____ means enlargement of the liver.

hepatitis   hepatomegaly   nephromegaly   nephritis

Challenge Word Building

These terms are *not* found in this chapter; however, they are made up of the following familiar word parts. If you need help in creating the term, refer to your medical dictionary.

neo- = new	arteri/o = artery	-algia = pain and suffering
	arthr/o = joint	-itis = inflammation
	cardi/o = heart	-ologist = specialist
	nat/o = birth	-otomy = a surgical incision
	neur/o = nerve	-rrhea = flow or discharge
	rhin/o = nose	-scopy = visual examination

1.86. A medical specialist concerned with the diagnosis and treatment of heart disease is a/an

_____ .

1.87. The term meaning a runny nose is _____ .

1.88. The term meaning the inflammation of a joint or joints is _____ .

1.89. A medical specialist in disorders of the newborn is a/an _____ .

1.90. The term meaning a surgical incision into a nerve is a/an _____ .

1.91. The term meaning the visual examination of the internal structure of a joint is _____ .

1.92. The term meaning pain in the nose is _____ .

1.93. The term meaning pain in a nerve or nerves is _____ .

1.94. The term meaning a surgical incision into the heart is a/an _____ .

1.95. The term meaning an inflammation of the nose is _____ .

Labeling Exercises

1.96. The combining form meaning spinal cord is

_____ / ___ .

1.97. The combining form meaning muscle is

_____ / ___ .

1.98. The combining form meaning bone marrow is

_____ / ___ .

1.99. The combining form meaning nerve is

_____ / ___ .

1.100. The combining form meaning joint is

_____ / ___ .

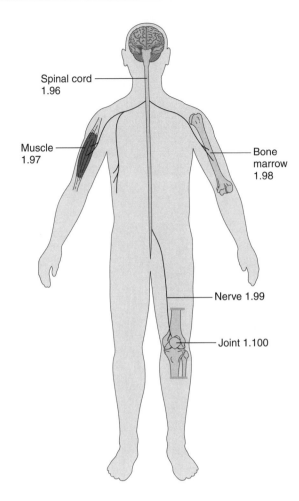

Spinal cord
1.96

Muscle
1.97

Bone
marrow
1.98

Nerve 1.99

Joint 1.100

The Human Body in Health and Disease

Learning Exercises

Class _____   Name _____

Matching Word Parts 1

Write the correct answer in the middle column.

Definition	Correct Answer	Possible Answers
2.1. fat	_____	aden/o
2.2. front	_____	adip/o
2.3. gland	_____	anter/o
2.4. specialist	_____	-ologist
2.5. study of	_____	-ology

Matching Word Parts 2

Write the correct answer in the middle column.

Definition	Correct Answer	Possible Answers
2.6. cell	_____	caud/o
2.7. head	_____	cephal/o
2.8. lower part of the body	_____	cyt/o
2.9. out of	_____	endo-
2.10. within	_____	exo-

Matching Word Parts 3
Write the correct answer in the middle column.

Definition	Correct Answer	Possible Answers
2.11. back	_____	hist/o
2.12. control	_____	path/o
2.13. disease, suffering, emotion	_____	-plasia
2.14. formation	_____	poster/o
2.15. tissue	_____	-stasis

Definitions
Select the correct answer and write it on the line provided.

2.16. A/An _____ _____ is acquired in a hospital setting.

    iatrogenic illness   idiopathic disease   nosocomial infection   organic disorder

2.17. When a _____ _____ is inherited from only one parent, the offspring will have that genetic condition or characteristic.

    dominant gene   genome   recessive gene   recessive trait

2.18. The _____ _____ contains the major organs of digestion.

    abdominal cavity   cranial cavity   dorsal cavity   pelvic cavity

2.19. The term _____ means the direction toward or nearer the midline.

    distal   lateral   medial   proximal

2.20. The primary role of the undifferentiated _____ _____ cells is to maintain and repair the tissue in which they are found.

    adult stem   cord blood   embryonic stem   hemopoietic

2.21. The genetic disorder _____ _____ is characterized by a missing digestive enzyme.

    Down syndrome   Huntington's disease   phenylketonuria   Tay-Sachs disease

2.22. The inflammation of a gland is known as _____ .

    adenectomy   adenitis   adenoma   adenosis

2.23. The _____ _____ is the outer layer of the peritoneum that lines the interior of the abdominal wall.

    mesentery   parietal peritoneum   retroperitoneum   visceral peritoneum

2.24. A _____ is fundamental physical and functional unit of heredity.

    cell   gamete   gene   genome

2.25. The study of the structure, composition, and function of tissues is known as _____ .

    anatomy   cytology   histology   physiology

Matching Regions of the Thorax and Abdomen

Write the correct answer in the middle column.

Definition	Correct Answer	Possible Answers
2.26. above the stomach	_____	epigastric region
2.27. belly button area	_____	hypochondriac region
2.28. below the ribs	_____	hypogastric region
2.29. below the stomach	_____	iliac region
2.30. hipbone area	_____	umbilicus region

Which Word?

Select the correct answer and write it on the line provided.

2.31. The term _____ refers to the entire lower portion of the abdomen.

   inguinal   umbilicus

2.32. The study of how traits are transferred from parents to their children and the role of genes in health and disease is known as _____ .

   cytology   genetics

2.33. A specialist in the study of the outbreaks of disease is a/an _____ .

   epidemiologist   pathologist

2.34. The _____ - _____ excrete their secretions through ducts.

   endocrine glands   exocrine glands

2.35. The location of the stomach is _____ to the diaphragm.

   inferior   superior

Spelling Counts

Find the misspelled word in each sentence. Then write that word, spelled correctly, on the line provided.

2.36. The mesantry is a fused double layer of the parietal peritoneum. _____

2.37. Hemaphilia is a group of hereditary bleeding disorders in which one of the factors needed to clot the blood is missing. _____

2.38. Hypretrophy is a general increase in the bulk of a body part or organ due to an increase in the size, but not in the number, of cells in the tissues. _____

2.39. The protective covering for all of the internal and external surfaces of the body is formed by epithealial tissues. _____

2.40. An abnomolly is any deviation from what is regarded as normal. _____

Matching Pathology of Tissue Formation

Write the correct answer in the middle column.

Definition	Correct Answer	Possible Answers
2.41. the abnormal development of tissues and cells	_____	anaplasia
2.42. a change in the structure of cells and in their orientation to each other	_____	aplasia
2.43. an abnormal increase in the number of normal cells in normal arrangement in a tissue	_____	dysplasia
2.44. incomplete development of an organ or tissue	_____	hyperplasia
2.45. the defective development or congenital absence of an organ or tissue	_____	hypoplasia

Term Selection

Select the correct answer and write it on the line provided.

2.46. The term meaning situated nearest the midline or beginning of a body structure is

_____ .

    distal   lateral   medial   proximal

2.47. The term meaning situated in the back is _____ .

    anterior   posterior   superior   ventral

2.48. The body is divided into anterior and posterior portions by the _____ plane.

    frontal   horizontal   sagittal   transverse

2.49. The body is divided into equal vertical left and right halves by the _____ plane.

    coronal   midsagittal   sagittal   transverse

2.50. Part of the elbow is formed by the _____ end of the humerus.

    distal   lateral   medial   proximal

Sentence Completion

Write the correct term on the line provided.

2.51. _____ _____ is a genetic abnormality that is associated with a characteristic facial appearance, cognitive impairment, and physical abnormalities such as heart valve disease.

2.52. The study of the functions of the structures of the body is known as _____ .

2.53. The heart and the lungs are surrounded and protected by the _____ cavity.

2.54. An unfavorable response to prescribed medical treatment, such as severe burns resulting from radiation therapy, is known as a/an _____ illness.

2.55. The genetic structures located within the nucleus of each cell are known as _____ . These structures are made up of the DNA molecules containing the body's genes.

Word Surgery

Divide each term into its component word parts. Write these word parts, in sequence, on the lines provided. When necessary use a slash (/) to indicate a combining vowel. (You may not need all of the lines provided.)

2.56. An **adenectomy** is the surgical removal of a gland.

_____   _____   _____   _____

2.57. Hormones are secreted directly into the bloodstream by the **endocrine** glands.

_____   _____   _____   _____

2.58. A **histologist** is a specialist in the study of the organization of tissues at all levels.

_____   _____   _____   _____

2.59. The term **retroperitoneal** means located behind the peritoneum.

_____   _____   _____   _____

2.60. A **pathologist** specializes in the laboratory analysis of tissue samples to confirm or establish a diagnosis.

_____   _____   _____   _____

2.61. The study of the causes of diseases is known as **etiology**.

_____   _____   _____   _____

2.62. The term **homeostasis** means maintaining a constant internal environment.

_____   _____   _____   _____

2.63. A **pandemic** is an outbreak of a disease occurring over a large geographic area, possibly worldwide.

_____   _____   _____   _____

2.64. The **epigastric** region is located above the stomach.

_____   _____   _____   _____

2.65. An **idiopathic** disorder is an illness without known cause.

_____   _____   _____   _____

Clinical Conditions

Write the correct answer on the line provided.

2.66. Mr. Tseng died of cholera during a sudden and widespread outbreak of this disease in his village. Such an outbreak is described as being a/an _____ .

2.67. Brenda Farmer's doctor could not find any physical changes to explain her symptoms. The doctor refers to this as a/an _____ disorder.

2.68. Gerald Carlson was infected with hepatitis B through _____ transmission.

2.69. In order to become a specialist in the structure and functions of cells, Lee Wong signed up for courses in _____ .

2.70. Malaria and the West Nile virus are spread by mosquitoes. This is known as _____-_____ transmission.

2.71. Jose Ortega complained of pain in the lower right area of his abdomen. Using the system that divides the abdomen into four sections, his doctor recorded the pain as being in the lower right _____ .

2.72. Ralph Jenkins was very sick after drinking contaminated water during a camping trip. His doctor says that he contracted the illness through _____ transmission.

2.73. Tracy Ames has a bladder inflammation. This organ of the urinary system is located in the _____ cavity.

2.74. Mrs. Reynolds was diagnosed as having inflammation of the peritoneum. The medical term for this condition is _____ .

2.75. Ashley Goldberg is fascinated by genetics. She wants to specialize in this field and is studying to become a/an _____ .

Which Is the Correct Medical Term?

Select the correct answer and write it on the line provided.

2.76. Debbie Sanchez fell against a rock and injured her left hip and upper leg. This area is known as the left _____ region.

   hypochondriac   iliac   lumbar   umbilical

2.77. A _____ is the complete set of genetic information of an individual.

   cell   gamete   gene   genome

2.78. An _____ is a malignant tumor that originates in glandular tissue.

   adenocarcinoma   adenitis   adenoma   adenosis

2.79. Nerve cells and blood vessels are surrounded and supported by _____ connective tissue.

   adipose   epithelial   liquid   loose

2.80. Maternal alcohol consumption during pregnancy can cause _____ _____ _____ .

   cerebral palsy   Down syndrome   fetal alcohol syndrome   genetic disorders

Challenge Word Building

These terms are *not* found in this chapter; however, they are made up of the following familiar word parts. If you need help in creating the term, refer to your medical dictionary.

   gastr/o = stomach   -algia = pain
   laryng/o = larynx   -ectomy = surgical removal
   my/o = muscle   -itis = inflammation
   nephr/o = kidney   -osis = abnormal condition or disease
   neur/o = nerve   -plasty = surgical repair

2.81. The term meaning the surgical repair of a muscle is _____ .

2.82. The term meaning muscle pain is _____ .

2.83. The term meaning an abnormal condition of the stomach is _____ .

2.84. The term meaning inflammation of the larynx is _____ .

2.85. The term meaning the surgical removal of part of a muscle is a/an _____ .

2.86. The term meaning pain in the stomach is _____ .

2.87. The term meaning surgical removal of the larynx is _____ .

2.88. The term meaning an abnormal condition of the kidney is _____ .

2.89. The medical term meaning surgical repair of a nerve is _____ .

2.90. The term meaning inflammation of the kidney is _____ .

Labeling Exercises

Identify the numbered items in the accompanying figures.

2.91. This is the right _____ region.

2.92. This is the _____ region.

2.93. This is the _____ region.

2.94. This is the left _____ region.

2.95. This is the left _____ region.

2.96. This is the _____ plane, which is also known as the midline.

2.97. This is the _____ surface, which is also known as the ventral surface.

2.98. This arrow is pointing in a/an

_____ direction.

2.99. This is the _____ surface, which is also known as the dorsal surface.

2.100. This is the _____ plane, which is also known as the coronal plane.

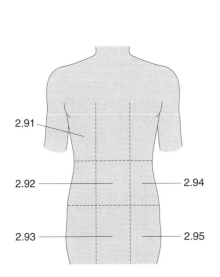

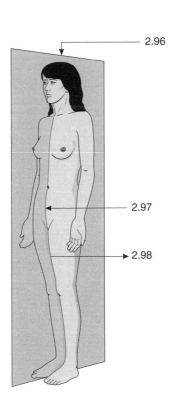

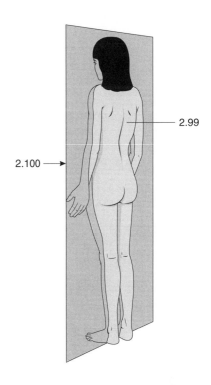

WORD PART REVIEW

In the first two chapters of your textbook, you were introduced to many word parts. The next 14 chapters cover the body systems. You will find that mastering this information is much easier if you have already learned *at least* the word parts in these first two chapters.

This special section, which is divided into two parts, is designed to reinforce your knowledge of these word parts and to confirm your mastery of them.

- The **Word Part Practice Session** includes 50 questions to provide additional word part practice, as well as opportunities to combine vowels correctly and build unfamiliar terms based on familiar word parts.

- The **Post-Test** that follows includes 50 questions designed to enable you to evaluate your mastery of these word parts. If you are having problems here, now is the time to ask your teacher for help.

WORD PART PRACTICE SESSION

Class _____   Name _____

Matching Prefixes #1
Write the correct answer in the middle column.

	Definition	Correct Answer	Possible Answers
WP.1.	bad, difficult, painful	_____	intra-
WP.2.	between, among	_____	hyper-
WP.3.	deficient, decreased	_____	inter-
WP.4.	excessive, increased	_____	hypo-
WP.5.	within, inside	_____	dys-

Matching Prefixes #2
Write the correct answer in the middle column.

	Definition	Correct Answer	Possible Answers
WP.6.	above, excessive	_____	pre-
WP.7.	before	_____	peri-
WP.8.	many	_____	poly-
WP.9.	surrounding	_____	sub-
WP.10.	under, less, below	_____	supra-

Matching Suffixes #1

Write the correct answer in the middle column.

Definition	Correct Answer	Possible Answers
WP.11. inflammation	_____	-algia
WP.12. pain, suffering	_____	-centesis
WP.13. the process of producing a picture or record	_____	-ectomy
WP.14. surgical puncture to remove fluid	_____	-itis
WP.15. surgical removal	_____	-graphy

Matching Suffixes #2

Write the correct answer in the middle column.

Definition	Correct Answer	Possible Answers
WP.16. surgical repair	_____	-dynia
WP.17. abnormal softening	_____	-malacia
WP.18. pain	_____	-necrosis
WP.19. tissue death	_____	-oma
WP.20. tumor or neoplasm	_____	-plasty

Matching Suffixes #3

Write the correct answer in the middle column.

Definition	Correct Answer	Possible Answers
WP.21. abnormal condition, disease	_____	-ac
WP.22. abnormal hardening	_____	-ostomy
WP.23. cutting, surgical incision	_____	-osis
WP.24. pertaining to	_____	-otomy
WP.25. surgical creation of an opening	_____	-sclerosis

Matching Suffixes #4

Write the correct answer in the middle column.

Definition	Correct Answer	Possible Answers
WP.26. abnormal flow, discharge	_____	-rrhagia
WP.27. abnormal tightening or narrowing	_____	-rrhaphy
WP.28. bleeding	_____	-rrhea
WP.29. rupture	_____	-rrhexis
WP.30. to suture	_____	-stenosis

True/False

If the statement is true, write **True** on the line. If the statement is false, write **False** on the line.

WP.31. _____ myc/o means mucous.

WP.32. _____ peri- means surrounding.

WP.33. _____ hyper- means below, under, decreased.

WP.34. _____ ather/o means plaque or fatty substance.

WP.35. _____ -gram means the process of producing a picture or record.

WP.36. _____ arthr/o means joint.

WP.37. _____ -ologist means study of.

WP.38. _____ -megaly means enlargement.

WP.39. _____ -centesis means to see or a visual examination.

Word Building

Write the word you created on the line provided.

WP.40. The term _____ means the surgical repair of the nose. (rhin/o means nose.)

WP.41. The term _____ means the surgical removal of a kidney. (nephr/o means kidney.)

WP.42. The term _____ means inflammation of the ear. (ot/o means ear.)

WP.43. The term _____ means an enlarged heart. (cardi/o means heart.)

WP.44. The term _____ means inflammation of the liver. (hepat/o means liver.)

WP.45. The term _____ means the visual examination of the interior of a joint. (arthr/o means joint.)

WP.46. A/An _____ is a specialist in disorders of the urinary system. (ur/o means urine.)

WP.47. The term _____ means the study of disorders of the blood. (hemat/o means blood.)

WP.48. The term _____ means a surgical incision into the colon. (col/o means colon.)

WP.49. The term _____ means inflammation of a vein. (phleb/o means vein.)

WP.50. The term _____ (ECG) means a record of the electrical activity of the heart. (electr/o means electric, and cardi/o means heart.)

WORD PART POST-TEST

Write the word part on the line provided.

PT.1. The suffix meaning surgical removal is _____ .

PT.2. The prefix meaning under, less, or below is _____ .

PT.3. The suffix meaning surgical repair is _____ .

PT.4. The combining form meaning fungus is _____ .

PT.5. The combining form meaning joint is _____ .

PT.6. The combining form meaning muscle is _____ .

PT.7. The prefix meaning between, among is _____ .

PT.8. The combining form meaning bone marrow *or* spinal cord is _____ .

PT.9. The suffix meaning to see or a visual examination is _____ .

PT.10. The suffix meaning the study of is _____ .

Matching Word Parts #1
Write the correct answer in the middle column.

Definition	Correct Answer	Possible Answers
PT.11. tumor	_____	arteri/o
PT.12. surgical suturing	_____	-oma
PT.13. surrounding	_____	peri-
PT.14. rupture	_____	-rrhaphy
PT.15. artery	_____	-rrhexis

Matching Word Parts #2
Write the correct answer in the middle column.

Definition	Correct Answer	Possible Answers
PT.16. abnormal hardening	_____	-itis
PT.17. bad, difficult, painful	_____	-ostomy
PT.18. inflammation	_____	-osis
PT.19. surgical creation of an opening	_____	dys-
PT.20. abnormal condition or disease	_____	-sclerosis

True/False
If the statement is true, write **True** on the line. If the statement is false, write **False** on the line.

PT.21. _____ The combining form hem/o means blood.

PT.22. _____ The suffix -algia means pain.

PT.23. _____ The combining form oste/o means bone.

PT.24. _____ The prefix hyper- means deficient or decreased.

PT.25. _____ The combining form rhin/o means nose.

PT.26. _____ Tonsillitis is an inflammation of the tonsils.

PT.27. _____ A myectomy is a surgical incision into a muscle.

PT.28. _____ Gastralgia is pain in the stomach.

PT.29. _____ A gerontologist specializes in the diseases of women.

PT.30. _____ The combining form cyan/o means gray.

Word Building
Write the word you created on the line provided.

Regarding Nerves (neur/o means nerve)

PT.31. A surgical incision into a nerve is a/an _____ .

PT.32. The study of the nervous system is known as _____ .

PT.33. The surgical repair of a nerve or nerves is a/an _____ .

PT.34. The term meaning to suture the ends of a severed nerve is _____ .

PT.35. Abnormal softening of the nerves is called _____ .

PT.36. A specialist in diagnosing and treating disorders of the nervous system is a/an
_____ .

PT.37. The term meaning inflammation of a nerve or nerves is _____ .

Relating to Blood Vessels (angi/o means relating to the blood vessels)

PT.38. The death of the walls of blood vessels is _____ .

PT.39. The abnormal hardening of the walls of blood vessels is _____ .

PT.40. The abnormal narrowing of a blood vessel is _____ .

PT.41. The surgical removal of a blood vessel is a/an _____ .

PT.42. The process of recording a picture of blood vessels is called _____ .

Missing Words

Write the missing word on the line provided.

PT.43. The surgical repair of an artery is a/an _____ . (arteri/o means artery.)

PT.44. The medical term meaning inflammation of the larynx is _____ . (laryng/o means larynx.)

PT.45. The surgical removal of all or part of the colon is a/an _____ . (col/o means colon.)

PT.46. The abnormal softening of muscle tissue is _____ . (my/o means muscle.)

PT.47. The term meaning any abnormal condition of the stomach is _____ . (gastr/o means stomach.)

PT.48. The term meaning the study of the heart is _____ . (cardi/o means heart.)

PT.49. The term meaning inflammation of the colon is _____ . (col/o means colon.)

PT.50. The term meaning a surgical incision into a vein is _____ . (phleb/o means vein.)

The Skeletal System

Learning Exercises

Class _____   Name _____

Matching Word Parts 1
Write the correct answer in the middle column.

Definition	Correct Answer	Possible Answers
3.1. hump	_____	ankyl/o
3.2. cartilage	_____	arthr/o
3.3. crooked, bent, or stiff	_____	-um
3.4. joint	_____	kyph/o
3.5. noun ending	_____	chondr/o

Matching Word Parts 2
Write the correct answer in the middle column.

Definition	Correct Answer	Possible Answers
3.6. cranium, skull	_____	cost/o
3.7. rib	_____	crani/o
3.8. setting free, loosening	_____	-desis
3.9. spinal cord, bone marrow	_____	-lysis
3.10. surgical fixation of a bone or joint	_____	myel/o

Matching Word Parts 3
Write the correct answer in the middle column.

Definition	Correct Answer	Possible Answers
3.11. vertebra, vertebrae	_____	oste/o
3.12. curved	_____	spondyl/o
3.13. bent backward	_____	lord/o
3.14. synovial membrane	_____	synovi/o, synov/o
3.15. bone	_____	scoli/o

Definitions

Select the correct answer and write it on the line provided.

3.16. The shaft of a long bone is known as the _____ _____ .

diaphysis   distal epiphysis   endosteum   proximal epiphysis

3.17. Seven short _____ bones make up each ankle.

carpal   metatarsal   phalanx   tarsal

3.18. The upper portion of the sternum is the _____ .

clavicle   mandible   manubrium   xiphoid process

3.19. A _____ _____ is movable.

cartilaginous joint   fibrous joint   suture joint   synovial joint

3.20. The _____ bone is located just below the urinary bladder.

ilium   ischium   pubis   sacrum

3.21. The opening in a bone through which the blood vessels, nerves, and ligaments pass

is a _____ .

foramen   foramina   process   symphysis

3.22. A/An _____ _____ connects one bone to another bone.

articular cartilage   ligament   synovial membrane   tendon

3.23. The hip socket is known as the _____ .

acetabulum   malleolus   patella   trochanter

3.24. The bones of the fingers and toes are known as the _____ .

carpals   metatarsals   tarsals   phalanges

3.25. A normal projection on the surface of a bone that serves as an attachment for muscles and tendons

is known as a/an _____ .

cruciate   exostosis   popliteal   process

Matching Structures

Write the correct answer in the middle column.

Definition	Correct Answer	Possible Answers
3.26. breastbone	_____	clavicle
3.27. cheekbones	_____	olecranon process
3.28. collarbone	_____	sternum
3.29. kneecap	_____	patella
3.30. point of the elbow	_____	zygomatic

Which Word?

Select the correct answer and write it on the line provided.

3.31. The surgical procedure for loosening of an ankylosed joint is known as _____ .

arthrodesis   arthrolysis

3.32. The bone disorder of unknown cause that destroys normal bone structure and replaces it with

fibrous (scar-like) tissue is known as _____ _____ .

fibrous dysplasia   Paget's disease

3.33. An _____ bone marrow transplant uses bone marrow from a donor.

allogenic   autologous

3.34. A percutaneous _____ is performed to treat osteoporosis related compression
fractures.

diskectomy   vertebroplasty

3.35. The medical term for the form of arthritis that is commonly known as wear-and-tear arthritis is

_____ .

osteoarthritis   rheumatoid arthritis

Spelling Counts

Find the misspelled word in each sentence. Then write that word, spelled correctly, on the line provided.

3.36. The medical term for the condition commonly known as low back pain is lumbaego.

_____

3.37. The surgical fracture of a bone to correct a deformity is known as osteclasis. _____

3.38. Ankylosing spondilitis is a form of rheumatoid arthritis characterized by progressive stiffening of the

spine. _____

3.39. An osterrhaphy is the surgical suturing, or wiring together, of bones. _____

3.40. Crepetation is the sound that is heard when the ends of a broken bone move together.

_____

Abbreviation Identification

Write the correct answer on the line provided.

3.41. **BMT** _____

3.42. **CR** _____

3.43. **Fx** _____

3.44. **RA** _____

3.45. **TMJ** _____

Term Selection

Select the correct answer and write it on the line provided.

3.46. The term meaning the death of bone tissue is _____ _____ .

osteitis deformans   osteomyelitis   osteonecrosis   osteoporosis

3.47. An abnormal increase in the forward curvature of the lower or lumbar spine is known as

_____ .

kyphosis   lordosis   scoliosis   spondylosis

3.48. The condition known as _____ _____ is a congenital defect.

juvenile arthritis   osteoarthritis   rheumatoid arthritis   spina bifida

3.49. A malignant tumor composed of cells derived from blood-forming tissues of the bone marrow is

known as a/an _____ _____ .

chondroma   Ewing's sarcoma   myeloma   osteochondroma

3.50. The bulging deposit that forms around the area of the break during the healing of a fractured bone

is a _____ .

callus   crepitation   crepitus   luxation

Sentence Completion
Write the correct term on the line provided.

3.51. A/An _____ is performed to treat a patient with craniostenosis or to relieve increased
intracranial pressure.

3.52. The partial displacement of a bone from its joint is known as _____ .

3.53. The procedure that stiffens a joint or joins several vertebrae is _____ . This is also
known as surgical ankylosis or fusion.

3.54. The surgical procedure to replace a joint with an artificial joint is known as _____ .

3.55. A medical term for the condition commonly known as a bunion is _____

_____ .

Word Surgery
Divide each term into its component word parts. Write these word parts, in sequence, on the lines provided.
When necessary use a slash (/) to indicate a combining vowel. (You may not need all of the lines provided.)

3.56. A **bursectomy** is the surgical removal of a bursa.

_____   _____   _____   _____

3.57. An **osteochondroma** is a benign bony projection covered with cartilage.

_____   _____   _____   _____

3.58. **Osteomalacia,** also known as adult rickets, is abnormal softening of bones in adults.

_____   _____   _____   _____

3.59. **Periostitis** is an inflammation of the periosteum.

_____   _____   _____   _____

3.60. **Spondylolisthesis** is the forward movement of the body of one of the lower lumbar vertebra on the
vertebra below it.

_____   _____   _____   _____

True/False
If the statement is true, write **True** on the line. If the statement is false, write **False** on the line.

3.61. _____ Osteopenia is thinner than average bone density. This term is used to describe the condition
of someone who does not yet have osteoporosis, but is at risk for developing it.

3.62. _____ Paget's disease is caused by a deficiency of calcium and vitamin D in early childhood.

3.63. _____ Costochondritis is an inflammation of the cartilage that connects a rib to the sternum.

3.64. _____ Dislocation is the partial displacement of a bone from its joint.

3.65. _____ Arthroscopic surgery is a minimally invasive procedure for the treatment of the interior of a joint.

Clinical Conditions

Write the correct answer on the line provided.

3.66. When Bobby Kuhn fell out of a tree, the bone in his arm was partially bent and partially broken. Dr. Grafton described this as a/an _____ fracture and told the family that this type of fracture occurs primarily in children.

3.67. Eduardo Sanchez was treated for an inflammation of the bone and bone marrow. The medical term for this condition is _____ .

3.68. Beth Hubert's breast cancer spread to her bones. These new sites are referred to as

_____ _____ _____ .

3.69. Mrs. Morton suffers from dowager's hump. The medical term for this abnormal curvature of the spine is _____ .

3.70. Henry Turner wears a brace to improve the impaired function of his leg. The medical term for this orthopedic appliance is a/an _____ .

3.71. As the result of a head injury in an auto accident, Cheng required a/an _____ to relieve the rapidly increasing intracranial pressure within his skull.

3.72. Mrs. Gilmer has leukemia and requires a bone marrow transplant. Part of the treatment was the harvesting of her bone marrow so she could receive it later as a/an _____ bone marrow transplant.

3.73. Betty Greene has been running for several years; however, now her knees hurt. Dr. Morita diagnosed her condition as _____ , which is an abnormal softening of the cartilage in these joints.

3.74. Patty Turner (age 7) has symptoms that include a skin rash, fever, slowed growth, fatigue, and swelling in the joints. She was diagnosed as having juvenile _____ arthritis.

3.75. Heather Lewis has a very sore shoulder. Dr. Plunkett diagnosed this as an inflammation of the bursa and said that Heather's condition is _____ .

Which Is the Correct Medical Term?

Select the correct answer and write it on the line provided.

3.76. Rodney Horner is being treated for a _____ fracture in which the ends of the bones were crushed together.

Colles'   comminuted   compound   spiral

3.77. Alex Jordan fell and injured her knee. Her doctor performed a/an _____ to surgically repair the damaged cartilage.

arthroplasty   chondritis   chondroplasty   osteoplasty

3.78. Mrs. Palmer is at high risk for osteoporosis. To obtain a definitive evaluation of the status of her bone density, Mrs. Palmer's physician ordered a/an _____ _____ _____ test.

dual x-ray absorptiometry   MRI   x-ray   ultrasonic bone density

3.79. In an effort to return a fractured bone to normal alignment, Dr. Wong ordered _____ _____ . This procedure exerts a pulling force on the distal end of the affected limb.

external fixation   immobilization   internal fixation   traction

3.80. Baby Juanita was treated for _____ , which is a congenital deformity of the foot involving the talus (ankle bones). Her family calls this condition clubfoot.

osteomalacia   rickets   scoliosis   talipes

Challenge Word Building

These terms are *not* found in this chapter; however, they are made up of the following familiar word parts. If you need help in creating the term, refer to your medical dictionary.

poly-	arthr/o	-ectomy
	chondr/o	-itis
	cost/o	-malacia
	crani/o	-otomy
	oste/o	-pathy
		-sclerosis

3.81. Abnormal hardening of bone is known as _____ .

3.82. The surgical removal of a rib or ribs is a/an _____ .

3.83. Any disease of cartilage is known as _____ .

3.84. A surgical incision into a joint is a/an _____ .

3.85. Inflammation of cartilage is known as _____ .

3.86. The surgical removal of a joint is a/an _____ .

3.87. Inflammation of more than one joint is known as _____ .

3.88. Any disease involving the bones and joints is known as _____ .

3.89. A surgical incision or division of a rib or ribs is a/an _____ .

3.90. Abnormal softening of the skull is known as _____ .

Labeling Exercises
Identify the numbered items on the accompanying figures.

3.91. _____ vertebrae

3.92. _____

3.93. _____

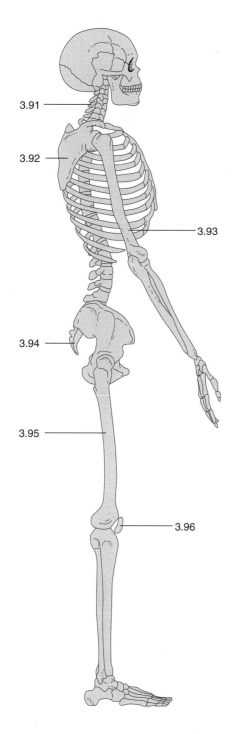

3.94. _____

3.95. _____

3.96. _____

3.97. _____ bone

3.98. _____ bone

3.99. _____ bone

3.100. _____

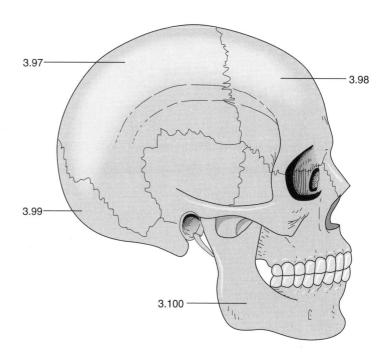

CHAPTER 4

The Muscular System

Learning Exercises

Class _____   Name _____

Matching Word Parts 1
Write the correct answer in the middle column.

Definition	Correct Answer	Possible Answers
4.1. condition	_____	-cele
4.2. fascia	_____	fasci/o
4.3. fibrous connective tissue	_____	fibr/o
4.4. hernia, swelling	_____	-ia
4.5. movement, motion	_____	kines/o, kinesi/o

Matching Word Parts 2
Write the correct answer in the middle column.

Definition	Correct Answer	Possible Answers
4.6. coordination	_____	my/o
4.7. muscle	_____	-rrhexis
4.8. rupture	_____	tax/o
4.9. tendon	_____	tend/o
4.10. tone	_____	ton/o

Matching Muscle Directions and Positions
Write the correct answer in the middle column.

Definition	Correct Answer	Possible Answers
4.11. cross-wise	_____	lateralis
4.12. ring-like	_____	oblique
4.13. slanted at an angle	_____	rectus
4.14. straight	_____	sphincter
4.15. toward the side	_____	transverse

Definitions
Select the correct answer and write it on the line provided.

4.16. The _____ muscles are under voluntary control.

   involuntary   nonstriated   skeletal   visceral

4.17. A/An _____ _____ is thickening on the surface of the calcaneus bone.

   heel spur   impingement syndrome   overuse injury   shin splint

4.18. Turning the hand so the palm is upward is called _____ .

   extension   flexion   pronation   supination

4.19. One of the symptoms of Parkinson's disease is _____ , which is extreme slowness of movement.

   bradykinesia   dyskinesia   hypotonia   myotonia

4.20. A/An _____ _____ is a physician who specializes in physical medicine and rehabilitation with the focus on restoring function.

   exercise physiologist   physiatrist   physiologist   rheumatologist

4.21. The term _____ _____ means pertaining to muscle tissue and fascia.

   aponeurosis   fibrous sheath   myocardium   myofascial

4.22. A/An _____ is a narrow band of nonelastic, fibrous tissue that attaches a muscle to bone.

   aponeurosis   fascia   ligament   tendon

4.23. A band of fibers that holds structures together abnormally is a/an _____ . These bands can form as the result of an injury or surgery.

   adhesion   aponeurosis   atrophy   contracture

4.24. The paralysis of both legs and the lower part of the body is known as _____ .

   hemiparesis   hemiplegia   paraplegia   quadriplegia

4.25. The medical term meaning pain in a tendon is _____ or tenalgia.

   tenodesis   tenodynia   tendinosis   tenolysis

Abbreviation Identification
Write the correct answer on the line provided.

4.26. **CTS**   _____

4.27. **DTR**   _____

4.28. **ROM**   _____

4.29. **RSD**   _____

4.30. **SCI**   _____

Which Word?

Select the correct answer and write it on the line provided.

4.31. An injury to the body of the muscle or the attachment of a tendon is known as a/an

_____ . These are usually associated with overuse injuries that involve a

stretched or torn muscle or tendon attachment.

sprain   strain

4.32. A _____ _____ _____ is a drug that

causes temporary muscle paralysis by blocking the transmission of nerve stimuli to the muscles.

neuromuscular blocker   skeletal muscle relaxant

4.33. The condition of abnormal muscle tone that results in impairment of voluntary muscle movement is

known as _____ .

dystaxia   dystonia

4.34. Inflamed and swollen tendons caught in the narrow space between the bones within the shoulder joint

cause the condition known as _____ _____ .

impingement syndrome   intermittent claudication

4.35. The study of the human factors that affect the design and operation of tools and the work environment

is known as _____ .

ergonomics   kinesiology

Spelling Counts

Find the misspelled word in each sentence. Then write that word, spelled correctly, on the line provided.

4.36. An antispasmydic is administered to suppress smooth muscle contractions of the stomach, intestine or

bladder. _____

4.37. The medical term for hiccups is singulutas. _____

4.38. Myasthenia gravias is a chronic autoimmune disease that affects the neuromuscular junction and

produces serious weakness of voluntary muscles. _____

4.39. A ganglian cyst is a harmless fluid-filled swelling that occurs most commonly on the outer surface of

the wrist. _____

4.40. Pronetion is the movement that turns the palm of the hand downward or backward.

_____

Term Selection

Select the correct answer and write it on the line provided.

4.41. The term _____ means the rupture of a muscle is.

myocele   myorrhaphy   myorrhexis   myotomy

4.42. The term meaning the breaking down of muscle tissue is _____ .

myoclonus   myolysis   myomalacia   myoparesis

4.43. The term _____ means abnormally decreased muscle function or activity.

hyperkinesia   hypertonia   hypokinesia   hypotonia

4.44. A/An _____ _____ injury can be a strain or tear on any of the three muscles that straighten the hip and bend the knee.

Achilles tendon   hamstring   myofascial   shin splint

4.45. The specialized soft tissue manipulation technique used to ease the pain of conditions such as fibromyalgia, movement restrictions, and temporomandibular joint disorders is known as

_____ _____ .

myofascial release   occupational therapy   RICE   therapeutic ultrasound

Sentence Completion

Write the correct term on the line provided.

4.46. The process of recording the strength of muscle contractions as the result of electrical stimulation is called _____ (EMG).

4.47. An inflammation of the tissues surrounding the elbow is known as _____ .

4.48. The debilitating chronic condition characterized by fatigue, diffuse and or specific muscle, joint, or bone pain, and a wide range of other symptoms is known as _____ syndrome (FMS).

4.49. The movement during which the knees or elbows are bent to decrease the angle of the joints is known as _____ .

4.50. An inflammation of the plantar fascia that causes foot or heel pain when walking or running is known as _____ .

4.51. Pain in the leg muscles that occurs during exercise and is relieved by rest is known as

_____ _____ . This condition is due to poor circulation and is associated with peripheral vascular disease.

4.52. The release of a tendon from adhesions is known as _____ . This procedure is the opposite of tenodesis.

4.53. A/An _____ is a physician who specializes in the diagnosis and treatment of arthritis and other diseases of the joints that are characterized by inflammation in the connective tissues.

4.54. A weakness or slight muscular paralysis is known as _____ .

4.55. A stiff neck due to spasmodic contraction of the neck muscles that pull the head toward the affected side is known as _____ _____ or wryneck.

Word Surgery

Divide each term into its component word parts. Write these word parts, in sequence, on the lines provided. When necessary, use a slash (/) to indicate a combining vowel. (You may not need all of the lines provided.)

4.56. **Electroneuromyography** is a procedure for testing and recording neuromuscular activity by the electric stimulation of the nerve trunk.

_____   _____   _____   _____

4.57. **Hyperkinesia** means abnormally increased motor function or activity.

_____   _____   _____   _____

4.58. **Myoclonus** is the sudden, involuntary jerking of a muscle or group of muscles.

_____   _____   _____   _____

4.59. **Polymyositis** is a muscle disease characterized by the inflammation and weakening of voluntary muscles in many parts of the body at the same time.

_____   _____   _____   _____

4.60. **Sarcopenia** is the age-related reduction in skeletal muscle mass in the elderly.

_____   _____   _____   _____

True/False

If the statement is true, write **True** on the line. If the statement is false, write **False** on the line.

4.61. _____ Overuse tendinitis is inflammation of tendons caused by excessive or unusual use of a joint.

4.62. _____ Hemiplegia is the total paralysis of the lower half of the body.

4.63. _____ A spasm is a sudden, violent, involuntary contraction of one or more muscles.

4.64. _____ Ataxia is the distortion of voluntary movement such as in a tic or spasm.

4.65. _____ Striated muscles are located in the walls of internal organs such as the digestive tract, blood vessels, and ducts leading from glands.

Clinical Conditions

Write the correct answer on the line provided.

4.66. George Quinton developed a swelling on the outer surface of his wrist. His doctor diagnosed this

as being a/an _____ _____ and explained that this was a harmless fluid-filled swelling.

4.67. Raul Valladares has a protrusion of a muscle substance through a tear in the fascia surrounding it. This

condition is known as a/an _____ .

4.68. Louisa Ferraro experienced _____ of her leg muscles due to the disuse of these muscles over a long period of time.

4.69. Jasmine Franklin has _____ . This is a condition in which there is diminished tone of the skeletal muscles.

4.70. Carolyn Goodwin complained of profound fatigue that is not improved by bed rest and was made worse by physical or mental activity. After ruling out other causes, her physician diagnosed her

condition as being _____ _____ syndrome (CFS).

4.71. Chuan Lee, who is a runner, required treatment for _____

_____ . This condition is a painful inflammation of the Achilles tendon caused by excessive stress being placed on that tendon.

4.72. For the first several days after his fall, Bob Hill suffered severe muscle pain. This condition is known

as _____ or myodynia.

4.73. Jose could not play for his team because of a/an _____ _____ . This is a painful condition caused by the muscle tearing away from the tibia.

4.74. Due to a spinal cord injury, Marissa Giannati suffers from _____ , which is paralysis of all four limbs.

4.75. Duncan McDougle has slight paralysis on one side of his body. This condition, which was caused by a

stroke, is known as _____ .

Which Is the Correct Medical Term?

Select the correct answer and write it on the line provided.

4.76. The term _____ describes a neuromuscular disorder characterized by the slow relaxation of the muscles after a voluntary contraction.

atonic   dystaxia   dystonia   myotonia

4.77. The term _____ , which is also known as tendinoplasty, is the surgical repair of a tendon.

tenectomy   tenodesis   tenolysis   tenoplasty

4.78. During _____ , the arm moves inward and toward the side of the body.

abduction   adduction   circumduction   rotation

4.79. Abnormal softening of a muscle is known as _____ .

myomalacia   myorrhaphy   myorrhexis   myosclerosis

4.80. The term _____ _____ means bending the foot upward at the ankle.

abduction   dorsiflexion   elevation   plantar flexion

Challenge Word Building

These terms are *not* found in this chapter; however, they are made up of the following familiar word parts. If you need help in creating the term, refer to your medical dictionary.

poly-	card/o	-algia
	fasci/o	-desis
	herni/o	-ectomy
	my/o	-itis
	sphincter/o	-necrosis
		-otomy
		-pathy
		-rrhaphy

4.81. Any abnormal condition of skeletal muscles is known as _____ .

4.82. Pain in several muscle groups is known as _____ .

4.83. The death of individual muscle fibers is known as _____ .

4.84. Surgical suturing of torn fascia is known as _____ .

4.85. A surgical incision into a muscle is a/an _____ .

4.86. The surgical attachment of a fascia to another fascia or to a tendon is known as

_____ .

4.87. Inflammation of the muscle of the heart is known as _____ .

4.88. The surgical removal of fascia is a/an _____ .

4.89. The surgical suturing of a defect in a muscular wall, such as the repair of a hernia, is a/an

_____ .

4.90. An incision into a sphincter muscle is a/an _____ .

Labeling Exercises

Identify the movements in the accompanying figures by writing the correct term on the line provided.

4.91. _____

4.92. _____

4.93. _____

4.94. _____

4.95. _____

4.96. _____

4.97. _____

4.98. _____

4.99. _____

4.100. _____

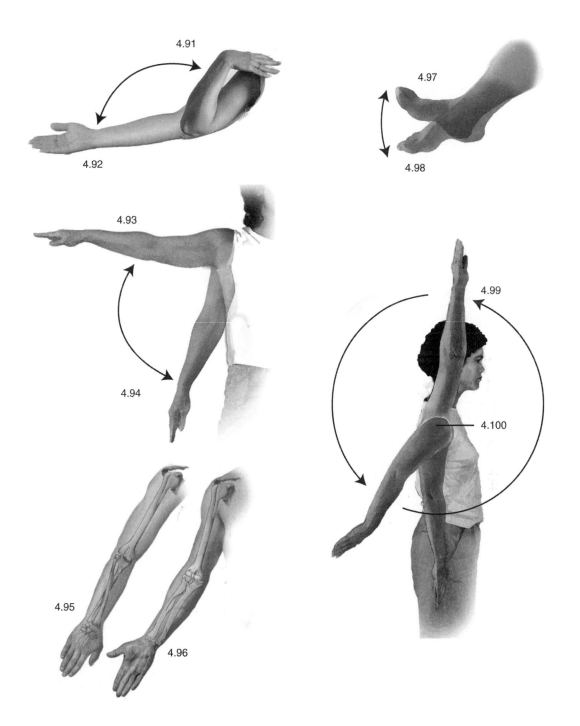

CHAPTER 5

The Cardiovascular System

Learning Exercises

Class _____   Name _____

Matching Word Parts 1
Write the correct answer in the middle column.

Definition	Correct Answer	Possible Answers
5.1. aorta	_____	angi/o
5.2. artery	_____	aort/o
5.3. plaque, fatty substance	_____	arteri/o
5.4. relating to blood or lymph vessels	_____	ather/o
5.5. slow	_____	brady-

Matching Word Parts 2
Write the correct answer in the middle column.

Definition	Correct Answer	Possible Answers
5.6. blood or blood condition	_____	cardi/o
5.7. heart	_____	-crasia
5.8. mixture or blending	_____	ven/o
5.9. red	_____	-emia
5.10. vein	_____	erythr/o

Matching Word Parts 3
Write the correct answer in the middle column.

Definition	Correct Answer	Possible Answers
5.11. white	_____	hem/o
5.12. vein	_____	leuk/o
5.13. fast, rapid	_____	phleb/o
5.14. clot	_____	tachy-
5.15. blood, relating to blood	_____	thromb/o

Definitions

Select the correct answer and write it on the line provided.

5.16. The term meaning white blood cells is _____ .

    erythrocytes   leukocytes   platelets   thrombocytes

5.17. Commonly known as the natural pacemaker, the medical name of the structure is the

_____ _____ _____ .

    atrioventricular node   bundle of His   Purkinje fiber   sinoatrial node

5.18. The myocardium receives its blood supply from the _____

_____ _____ .

    aorta   coronary arteries   inferior vena cava   superior vena cava

5.19. The _____ are formed in red bone marrow and then migrate to tissues throughout the body. These blood cells destroy parasitic organisms and play a major role in allergic reactions.

    basophils   eosinophils   erythrocytes   monocytes

5.20. The bicuspid heart valve is also known as the _____ valve.

    aortic   mitral   pulmonary   tricuspid

5.21. The _____ _____ pumps blood into the pulmonary artery, which carries it to the lungs.

    left atrium   left ventricle   right atrium   right ventricle

5.22. The _____ are the smallest formed elements in the blood, and they play an important role in blood clotting.

    erythrocytes   leukocytes   monocytes   thrombocytes

5.23. A foreign object, such as a bit of tissue or air, circulating in the blood is known as a/an

_____ .

    embolism   embolus   thrombosis   thrombus

5.24. The _____ _____ carries blood to all parts of the body except the lungs.

    left atrium   left ventricle   right atrium   right ventricle

5.25. The _____ are the most common type of white blood cell.

    erythrocytes   leukocytes   neutrophils   thrombocytes

Matching Structures

Write the correct answer in the middle column.

Definition	Correct Answer	Possible Answers
5.26. a hollow, muscular organ	_____	endocardium
5.27. cardiac muscle	_____	epicardium
5.28. external layer of the heart	_____	heart
5.29. inner lining of the heart	_____	myocardium
5.30. sac enclosing the heart	_____	pericardium

Which Word?

Select the correct answer and write it on the line provided.

5.31. High-density _____ _____ is also known as good cholesterol.

lipoprotein cholesterol   total cholesterol

5.32. An abnormally slow resting heart rate is described as _____ .

bradycardia   tachycardia

5.33. In _____ fibrillation, instead of pumping strongly, the heart muscle quivers ineffectively.

atrial   ventricular

5.34. The highest pressure against the blood vessels is _____ pressure, and it occurs when the ventricles contract.

diastolic   systolic

5.35. The diagnostic procedure that images the structures of the blood vessels and the flow of blood through these vessels is known as _____ _____ .

digital angiography   duplex ultrasound

Spelling Counts

Find the misspelled word in each sentence. Then write that word, spelled correctly, on the line provided.

5.36. The autopsy indicated that the cause of death was a ruptured aneuryism. _____

5.37. A deficiency of blood passing through an organ or body part is known as hypoprefusion.

_____

5.38. An arrhythemia is an abnormal heart rhythm in which the heartbeat is faster, or slower than normal.

_____ .

5.39. Raynoud's phenomenon is a condition with symptoms that include of intermittent attacks of pallor, cyanosis, and redness of the fingers and toes. _____

5.40. An implantable cardiovarter defibrillator is a double-action pacemaker. _____

Abbreviation Identification

In the space provided, write the words that each abbreviation stands for.

5.41. **CAD**   _____

5.42. **EKG, ECG** _____

5.43. **Hb** or **HB** _____

5.44. **MI**   _____

5.45. **VF**   _____

Term Selection

Select the correct answer and write it on the line provided.

5.46.   The systemic condition caused by the spread of microorganisms and their toxins via the circulating blood is known as _____ .

dyscrasia   endocarditis   pericarditis   septicemia

5.47.   A/An _____-_____ reduces the workload of the heart by slowing the rate of the heartbeat.

ACE inhibitor   beta-blocker   calcium blocker   statin inhibitor

5.48.   The blood disorder characterized by anemia in which the red blood cells are larger than normal is known as _____ anemia.

aplastic   hemolytic   megaloblastic   pernicious

5.49.   A/An _____ is administered to lower high blood pressure.

antiarrhythmic   antihypertensive   digitalis   diuretic

5.50.   A bacterial infection of the lining or valves of the heart is known as bacterial

_____ .

endocarditis   myocarditis   pericarditis   valvulitis

Sentence Completion

Write the correct term on the line provided.

5.51.   Plasma with the clotting proteins removed is known as _____ .

5.52.   Having an abnormally small number of platelets in the circulating blood is known as

_____ .

5.53.   The surgical removal of the lining of a portion of a clogged carotid artery leading to the brain is known as a/an _____ _____ .

5.54.   The abnormal protrusion of a heart valve that results in the inability of the valve to close completely is known as a/an _____ .

5.55.   The medication _____ is prescribed to prevent or relieve the pain of angina by relaxing the blood vessels to the heart.

Word Surgery

Divide each term into its component word parts. Write these word parts, in sequence, on the lines provided. When necessary use a slash (/) to indicate a combining vowel. (You may not need all of the lines provided.)

5.56.   **Aneurysmorrhaphy** means the surgical suturing a ruptured aneurysm.

_____   _____   _____   _____

5.57.   **Aplastic** anemia is characterized by an absence of *all* formed blood elements.

_____   _____   _____   _____

5.58.   **Electrocardiography** is the process of recording the electrical activity of the myocardium.

_____   _____   _____   _____

5.59. **Polyarteritis** is a form of angiitis involving several medium and small arteries at the same time.

_____   _____   _____   _____

5.60. **Valvoplasty** is the surgical repair or replacement of a heart valve.

_____   _____   _____   _____

True/False

If the statement is true, write **True** on the line. If the statement is false, write **False** on the line.

5.61. _____ A thrombus is a clot or piece of tissue circulating in the blood.

5.62. _____ Hemochromatosis is also known as iron overload disease.

5.63. _____ Plasmapheresis is the removal of whole blood from the body, separation of its cellular elements, and reinfusion of these cellular elements suspended in saline or a plasma substitute.

5.64. _____ A vasoconstrictor is a drug that enlarges the blood vessels.

5.65. _____ Peripheral vascular disease is a disorder of the blood vessels located outside the heart and brain.

Clinical Conditions

Write the correct answer on the line provided.

5.66. Alberta Fleetwood has a/an _____ . This condition is a benign tumor made up of newly formed blood vessels.

5.67. After his surgery, Ramon Martinez developed a deep vein _____ (DVT) in his leg.

5.68. During her pregnancy, Polly Olson suffered from abnormally swollen veins in her legs. The medical term for this condition is _____ veins.

5.69. Thomas Wilkerson suffers from episodes of severe chest pain due to inadequate blood flow to the myocardium. This is a condition is known as _____ .

5.70. When Mr. Klein stands up too quickly, his blood pressure drops. His physician describes this as postural or _____ _____ .

5.71. Juanita Gomez was diagnosed as having _____ _____ . This cancerous blood condition was previously known as preleukemia.

5.72. Dr. Lawson read her patient's _____ . This diagnostic record is also known as an ECG or EKG.

5.73. Jason Turner suffered from cardiac arrest. The paramedics arrived promptly and saved his life by using _____ _____ (CPR).

5.74. Darlene Nolan was diagnosed as having a deep vein thrombosis. Her doctor immediately prescribed a/an _____ to cause the thrombus to dissolve.

5.75. Hamilton Edwards Sr. suffers from _____ heart disease (IHD). This is a group of cardiac disabilities resulting from an insufficient supply of oxygenated blood to the heart.

Which Is the Correct Medical Term?

Select the correct answer and write it on the line provided.

5.76. A/An _____ , which is a characteristic of atherosclerosis, is a deposit of plaque on or within the arterial wall.

    angiitis   angiostenosis   arteriosclerosis   atheroma

5.77. The term _____ means to stop or control bleeding.

    hemochromatosis   hemostasis   plasmapheresis   transfusion reaction

5.78. Inflammation of a vein is known as _____ .

    angiitis   arteritis   phlebitis   phlebostenosis

5.79. Blood _____ is any pathologic condition of the cellular elements of the blood.

    anemia   dyscrasia   hemochromatosis   septicemia

5.80. The surgical removal of an aneurysm is a/an _____ .

    aneurysmectomy   aneurysmoplasty   aneurysmorrhaphy   aneurysmotomy

Challenge Word Building

These terms are *not* found in this chapter; however, they are made up of the following familiar word parts. If you need help in creating the term, refer to your medical dictionary.

peri-	angi/o	-ectomy
	arter/o	-itis
	cardi/o	-necrosis
	phleb/o	-rrhaphy
		-rrhexis
		-stenosis

5.81. Inflammation of an artery or arteries is known as _____ .

5.82. The surgical removal of a portion of a blood vessel is a/an _____ .

5.83. The abnormal narrowing of the lumen of a vein is known as _____ .

5.84. The surgical removal of a portion of the tissue surrounding the heart is a/an _____ .

5.85. To surgically suture the wall of the heart is a/an _____ .

5.86. Rupture of a vein is known as _____ .

5.87. The suture repair of any vessel, especially a blood vessel, is a/an _____ .

5.88. Rupture of the heart is known as _____ .

5.89. To suture the tissue surrounding the heart is a/an _____ .

5.90. The tissue death of the walls of the blood vessels is known as _____ .

Labeling Exercises

Identify the numbered items in the accompanying figures.

5.91. Superior _____ _____

5.92. Right _____

5.93. Right _____

5.94. Left pulmonary _____

5.95. Left pulmonary _____

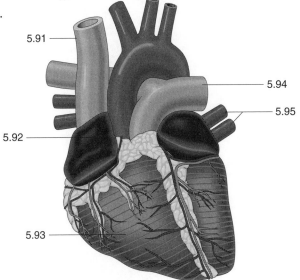

5.96. Pulmonary _____ valve

5.97. _____ valve

5.98. _____

5.99. _____ semilunar valve

5.100. _____ valve

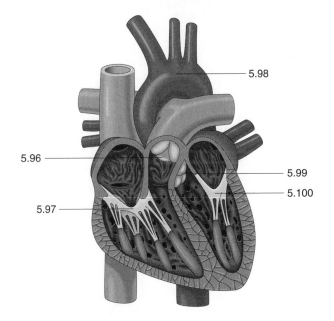

CHAPTER 6

The Lymphatic and Immune Systems

Learning Exercises

Class _____ Name _____

Matching Word Parts 1
Write the correct answer in the middle column.

Definition	Correct Answer	Possible Answers
6.1. against	_____	anti-
6.2. eat, swallow	_____	lymphaden/o
6.3. lymph node	_____	lymphangi/o
6.4. lymph vessel	_____	phag/o
6.5. poison	_____	tox/o

Matching Word Parts 2
Write the correct answer in the middle column.

Definition	Correct Answer	Possible Answers
6.6. flesh	_____	immun/o
6.7. formation	_____	onc/o
6.8. protected, safe	_____	-plasm
6.9. spleen	_____	sarc/o
6.10. tumor	_____	splen/o

Matching Types of Pathogens

Write the correct answer in the middle column.

Definition	Correct Answer	Possible Answers
6.11. bacteria capable of movement	_____	parasites
6.12. chain-forming bacteria	_____	spirochetes
6.13. cluster-forming bacteria	_____	staphylococci
6.14. live only by invading cells	_____	streptococci
6.15. live within other organisms	_____	viruses

Definitions

Select the correct answer and write it on the line provided.

6.16. The _____ _____ has/have a hemolytic function.

      appendix   lymph nodes   spleen   tonsils

6.17. Inflammation of the lymph nodes is known as _____ .

      adenoiditis   lymphadenitis   lymphedema   tonsillitis

6.18. The medical term for the condition is commonly known as shingles is _____

      _____ .

      cytomegalovirus   herpes zoster   rubella   varicella

6.19. The family of proteins whose specialty is fighting viruses by slowing or stopping their multiplication is

      known as _____ _____ .

      complement   immunoglobulin   interferon   synthetic immunoglobulin

6.20. The _____ _____ plays important roles in both the immune
and endocrine systems.

      bone marrow   liver   spleen   thymus

6.21. The protective ring of lymphoid tissue surrounding the internal openings of the nose and mouth is

      formed by the _____ _____ .

      lacteals   lymph nodes   tonsils   villi

6.22. Secondary _____ can be caused by cancer treatments, burns, or trauma.

      lymphadenitis   lymphangioma   lymphadenopathy   lymphedema

6.23. Fats and fat-soluble vitamins are absorbed by the _____ _____
that are located in the villi that line the small intestine.

      lacteals   lymph nodes   Peyer's patches   spleen

6.24. The parasite _____ _____ is most commonly transmitted from
pets to humans by contact with contaminated feces.

      herpes zoster   malaria   rabies   toxoplasmosis

6.25. A/An _____ is a type of white blood cell that surrounds and kills invading cells.
This type of cell also removes dead cells and stimulates the action of other immune cells.

      B lymphocyte   macrophage   platelet   T lymphocyte

Matching Structures

Write the correct answer in the middle column.

Definition	Correct Answer	Possible Answers
6.26. filter harmful substances from lymph	_____	complement
6.27. lymphoid tissue hanging from the lower portion of the cecum	_____	intact skin
6.28. marks foreign invaders and attracts phagocytes	_____	lymph nodes
6.29. stores extra erythrocytes	_____	spleen
6.30. wraps the body in a physical barrier	_____	vermiform appendix

Which Word?

Select the correct answer and write it on the line provided.

6.31. The _____ direct the antigen-antibody response by signaling between the cells of the immune system.

    lymphokines   macrophages

6.32. A _____ drug is a medication that kills or damages cells.

    corticosteroid   cytotoxic

6.33. The _____ _____ are specialized white blood cells that produce antibodies coded to destroy specific antigens.

    complement cells   plasma cells

6.34. The antibody therapy known as _____ _____ is used to treat multiple sclerosis, hepatitis C, and some cancers.

    monoclonal antibodies   synthetic interferon

6.35. Infectious mononucleosis is caused by a _____ .

    spirochete   virus

Spelling Counts

Find the misspelled word in each sentence. Then write that word, spelled correctly, on the line provided.

6.36. A sarkoma is a malignant tumor that arises from connective tissue. _____

6.37. The adenods, which are also known as the nasopharyngeal tonsils, are located in the nasopharynx. _____

6.38. Lymphangiscintigraphy is a diagnostic test that is performed to detect damage or malformations of the lymphatic vessels. _____

6.39. Antiobiotics are commonly used to combat bacterial infections. _____

6.40. Varizella is commonly known as chickenpox. _____

Abbreviation Identification
In the space provided, write the words that each abbreviation stands for.

6.41. **CIS** _____

6.42. **DCIS** _____

6.43. **LE** _____

6.44. **MMR** _____

6.45. **Rick** _____

Term Selection
Select the correct answer and write it on the line provided.

6.46. A/An _____ _____ is not life-threatening and not recurring.

   benign tumor   carcinoma in situ   invasive neoplasm   malignant tumor

6.47. An opportunistic infection commonly associated with HIV is _____

   _____ .

   Hodgkin's disease   Kaposi's sarcoma   myasthenia gravis   tinea pedis

6.48. Malaria is caused by a _____ that is transferred to humans by the bite of an infected mosquito.

   parasite   rickettsiae   spirochete   virus

6.49. Bacilli, which are rod-shaped spore-forming bacteria, cause _____ .

   Lyme disease   measles   rubella   tetanus

6.50. Swelling of the parotid glands is a symptom of _____ .

   measles   mumps   shingles   rubella

Sentence Completion
Write the correct term on the line provided.

6.51. A severe systemic reaction to a foreign substance causing serious symptoms that develop very quickly
   is known as _____ .

6.52. In _____ , radioactive materials are implanted into the tissues to be treated.

6.53. When testing for HIV, a/an _____ _____ test produces more
   accurate results than the ELISA test.

6.54. A/An _____ is a benign tumor formed by an abnormal collection of lymphatic
   vessels.

6.55. After primary cancer treatments have been completed, _____ therapy is used to
   decrease the chances that the cancer will recur.

Word Surgery

Divide each term into its component word parts. Write these word parts, in sequence, on the lines provided. When necessary, use a slash (/) to indicate a combining vowel. (You may not need all of the lines provided.)

6.56. An **antineoplastic** is a medication that blocks the development, growth, or proliferation of malignant cells.

_____ _____ _____ _____

6.57. **Metastasis** is the term describing the new site that results from the spreading of a cancer process.

_____ _____ _____ _____

6.58. **Osteosarcoma** is a malignant tumor usually involving the upper shaft of long bones, the pelvis, or knee.

_____ _____ _____ _____

6.59. **Cytomegalovirus** is a member of the herpesvirus family that cause a variety of diseases.

_____ _____ _____ _____

6.60. **Antiangiogenesis** is a form of cancer treatment that cuts off the blood supply to the tumor.

_____ _____ _____ _____

True/False

If the statement is true, write **True** on the line. If the statement is false, write **False** on the line.

6.61. _____ Inflammatory breast cancer is the most aggressive, and least familiar, form of breast cancer.

6.62. _____ Lymph carries nutrients and oxygen to the cells.

6.63. _____ A myosarcoma is a benign tumor derived from muscle tissue.

6.64. _____ Reed-Sternberg cells are present in Hodgkin's lymphoma.

6.65. _____ Septic shock is caused by a viral infection.

Clinical Conditions

Write the correct answer on the line provided.

6.66. Dr. Wei diagnosed her patient as having an enlarged spleen due to damage caused by his injuries.

The medical term for this condition is _____ .

6.67. At the beginning of the treatment of Juanita's breast cancer, a/an _____ node biopsy was performed.

6.68. Mr. Grossman described his serious illness as being caused by a "superbug infection." His doctor

describes these bacteria as being _____ _____ .

6.69. Dorothy Peterson was diagnosed with breast cancer. She and her doctor agreed upon treating this

surgically with a/an _____ . This is a procedure in which the tumor and a margin of healthy tissue are removed.

6.70. Every day since his kidney transplant, Mr. Lanning must take a/an _____ to prevent rejection of the donor organ.

6.71. Rosita Sanchez is 2 months pregnant, and she and her doctor are worried because her rash was

diagnosed as _____ . They are concerned because this condition can produce defects in Rosita's developing child.

6.72. Tarana Inglis took _____ to relieve the symptoms of her allergies.

6.73. The _____ _____ virus is carried by birds and transmitted to humans through the bites of mosquito or tick. If untreated, the inflammation can spread to the spinal cord and brain.

6.74. John Fogelman was diagnosed with having a/an _____ . This is a malignant tumor that arises from connective tissues, including hard tissues, soft tissues, and liquid tissues.

6.75. Jane Doe is infected with HIV. One of her medications is acyclovir, which is a/an

_____ drug.

Which Is the Correct Medical Term?

Select the correct answer and write it on the line provided.

6.76. _____ , also known as *B lymphocytes,* are specialized lymphocytes that produce and secrete antibodies. Each lymphocyte makes a specific antibody that is capable of destroying a specific antigen.

B cells	complement	immunoglobulins	T cells

6.77. _____ _____ is an autoimmune disorder.

Graves' disease	mumps	rubella	secondary lymphedema

6.78. The _____ lymph nodes are located in the groin.

axillary	cervical	inguinal	subcutaneous

6.79. A/An _____ is any one of a large group of carcinomas derived from glandular tissue.

adenocarcinoma	lymphoma	myosarcoma	myoma

6.80. A/An _____ _____ drug is used either as an immunosuppressant or as an antineoplastic.

corticosteroid	cytotoxic	immunoglobulin	monoclonal

Challenge Word Building

These terms are *not* found in this chapter; however, they are made up of the following familiar word parts. If you need help in creating the term, refer to your medical dictionary.

adenoid/o	-ectomy
lymphaden/o	-it is
lymphang/o	-ology
immun/o	-oma
splen/o	-rrhaphy
tonsill/o	
thym/o	

6.81. The study of the immune system is known as _____ .

6.82. Surgical removal of the spleen is a/an _____ .

6.83. Inflammation of the thymus is known as _____ .

6.84. Inflammation of the lymph vessels is known as _____ .

6.85. The term meaning to suture the spleen is _____ .

6.86. The surgical removal of the adenoids is a/an _____ .

6.87. The surgical removal of a lymph node is a/an _____ .

6.88. A tumor originating in the thymus is known as _____ .

6.89. Inflammation of the tonsils is known as _____ .

6.90. Inflammation of the spleen is known as _____ .

Labeling Exercises

Identify the numbered items on the accompanying figures.

6.91. tonsils and _____

6.92. Lymphocytes are formed in bone _____

6.93. appendix and _____ _____

6.94. _____

6.95. _____

6.96. _____ lymph nodes

6.97. Right _____ vein

6.98. _____ duct

6.99. _____ lymph nodes

6.100. _____ lymph nodes

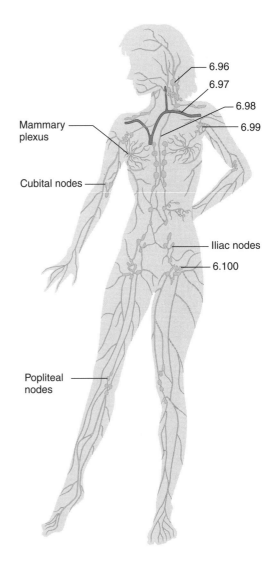

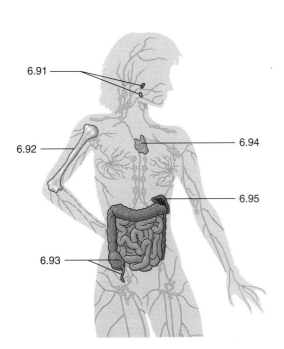

CHAPTER 7

The Respiratory System

Learning Exercises

Class _____   Name _____

Matching Word Parts 1

Write the correct answer in the middle column.

Definition	Correct Answer	Possible Answers
7.1. blue	_____	cyan/o
7.2. sleep	_____	laryng/o
7.3. to breathe	_____	pharyng/o
7.4. throat	_____	somn/o
7.5. voice box	_____	spir/o

Matching Word Parts 2

Write the correct answer in the middle column.

Definition	Correct Answer	Possible Answers
7.6. lung	_____	bronch/o
7.7. oxygen	_____	ox/o
7.8. multilayered membrane	_____	phon/o
7.9. bronchus	_____	pleur/o
7.10. voice or sound	_____	pneum/o

Matching Word Parts 3

Write the correct answer in the middle column.

Definition	Correct Answer	Possible Answers
7.11. windpipe	_____	-pnea
7.12. rapid	_____	pulmon/o
7.13. lung	_____	tachy-
7.14. chest	_____	-thorax
7.15. breathing	_____	trache/o

Definitions

Select the correct answer and write it on the line provided.

7.16. The heart, aorta, esophagus, and trachea are located in the _____

_____ .

dorsal cavity   manubrium   mediastinum   pleura

7.17. The _____ _____ acts as a lid over the entrance to the esophagus.

Adam's apple   epiglottis   larynx   thyroid cartilage

7.18. The innermost layer of the pleura is known as the _____ _____ .

parietal pleura   pleural space   pleural cavity   visceral pleura

7.19. The _____ sinuses are located just above the eyes.

ethmoid   frontal   maxillary   sphenoid

7.20. The smallest divisions of the bronchial tree are the _____ .

alveoli   alveolus   bronchioles   bronchi

7.21. During respiration, the exchange of gases takes place through the walls of the _____ .

alveoli   arteries   capillaries   veins

7.22. The term meaning spitting blood or blood-stained sputum is _____ .

effusion   epistaxis   hemoptysis   hemothorax

7.23. Black lung disease is the lay term for _____ .

anthracosis   byssinosis   pneumoconiosis   silicosis

7.24. The term _____ means an abnormally rapid rate of respiration.

apnea   bradypnea   dyspnea   tachypnea

7.25. The term meaning any voice impairment is _____ .

aphonia   dysphonia   laryngitis   laryngoplegia

Matching Structures

Write the correct answer in the middle column.

Definition	Correct Answer	Possible Answers
7.26. first division of the pharynx	_____	laryngopharynx
7.27. second division of the pharynx	_____	larynx
7.28. third division of the pharynx	_____	nasopharynx
7.29. voice box	_____	oropharynx
7.30. windpipe	_____	trachea

Which Word?

Select the correct answer and write it on the line provided.

7.31. The exchange of gases within the cells of the body is known as _____

_____ .

external respiration   internal respiration

7.32. The term that describes the lung disease caused by cotton dust is _____ .

byssinosis   silicosis

7.33. The form of pneumonia that can be prevented through vaccination is _____

_____ .

bacterial pneumonia   viral pneumonia

7.34. The term commonly known as shortness of breath is _____ .

dyspnea   eupnea

7.35. The emergency procedure to gain access below a blocked airway is known as a _____ .

tracheostomy   tracheotomy

Spelling Counts

Find the misspelled word in each sentence. Then write the word, spelled correctly, on the line provided.

7.36. The thick mucus secreted by the tissues that line the respiratory passages is called flem.

_____

7.37. The medical term meaning an accumulation of pus in the pleural cavity is emphyema.

_____

7.38. The medical name for the disease commonly known as whooping cough is pertussosis.

_____

7.39. The frenic nerve stimulates the diaphragm and causes it to contract. _____

7.40. An antitussiff is administered to prevent or relieve coughing. _____

Abbreviation Identification

In the space provided, write the words that each abbreviation stands for.

7.41. **ARDS** _____

7.42. **CF** _____

7.43. **FESS** _____

7.44. **SIDS** _____

7.45. **URI** _____

Term Selection

Select the correct answer and write it on the line provided.

7.46. Inhaling a foreign substance into the upper respiratory tract can cause _____ pneumonia.

aspiration   inhalation   inspiration   respiration

7.47. The term meaning abnormally rapid deep breathing _____ .

dyspnea   hyperpnea   hypopnea   hyperventilation

7.48. The term meaning the surgical repair of the trachea is _____ .

pharyngoplasty   tracheoplasty   tracheostomy   tracheotomy

7.49. The diaphragm is relaxed during _____ _____ .

    exhalation   inhalation   internal respiration   singultus

7.50. The chronic allergic disorder characterized by episodes of severe breathing difficulty, coughing, and wheezing is known as _____ _____ .

    allergic rhinitis   asthma   bronchospasm   laryngospasm

Sentence Completion

Write the correct term on the line provided.

7.51. The term meaning an absence of spontaneous respiration is _____ .

7.52. The sudden spasmodic closure of the larynx is a/an _____ .

7.53. The term meaning bleeding from the lungs is _____ .

7.54. The term meaning pain in the pleura or in the side is _____ .

7.55. A contraction of the smooth muscle in the walls of the bronchi and bronchioles that tighten and squeeze the airway shut is known as a/an _____ .

Word Surgery

Divide each term into its component word parts. Write these word parts, in sequence, on the lines provided. When necessary use a slash (/) to indicate a combining vowel. (You may not need all of the lines provided.)

7.56. **Bronchorrhea** means an excessive discharge of mucus from the bronchi.

_____ _____ _____ _____

7.57. The **oropharynx** is visible when looking at the back of the mouth.

_____ _____ _____ _____

7.58. **Polysomnography** measures physiological activity during sleep and is most often performed to detect nocturnal defects in breathing associated with sleep apnea.

_____ _____ _____ _____

7.59. **Pneumorrhagia** is bleeding from the lungs.

_____ _____ _____ _____

7.60. **Rhinorrhea,** also known as a runny nose, is an excessive flow of mucus from the nose.

_____ _____ _____ _____

True/False

If the statement is true, write **True** on the line. If the statement is false, write **False** on the line.

7.61. _____ A pulse oximeter is a monitor placed in the ear to measure the oxygen saturation level in the blood.

7.62. _____ In atelectasis, the lung fails to expand because air cannot pass beyond the bronchioles that are blocked by secretions.

7.63. _____ Croup is an allergic reaction to airborne allergens.

7.64. _____ Hypoxemia is the condition of below-normal oxygenation of arterial blood.

7.65. _____ Emphysema is the progressive loss of lung function in which the chest sometimes assumes an enlarged barrel shape.

Clinical Conditions

Write the correct answer on the line provided.

7.66. Baby Jamison was born with _____ _____ (CF). This is a genetic disorder in which the lungs are clogged with large quantities of abnormally thick mucus.

7.67. Dr. Lee surgically removed a portion of the pleura. This procedure is known as a/an

_____ .

7.68. Wendy Barlow required the surgical repair of her larynx. This procedure is known as a/an

_____ .

7.69. During his asthma attacks, Jamaal uses an inhaler containing a _____ . This medication expands the opening of the passages into his lungs.

7.70. Each year, Mr. Partin receives a flu shot to prevent _____ .

7.71. When hit during a fight, Marvin Roper's nose started to bleed. The medical term for this condition is

_____ .

7.72. The doctor's examination revealed that Juanita Martinez has an accumulation of blood in the pleural

cavity. This diagnosis is recorded on her chart as a/an _____ .

7.73. Duncan McClanahan had a/an _____ performed to correct damage to the septum of his nose.

7.74. Suzanne Holderman is suffering from an inflammation of the bronchial walls. The medical term for

Suzanne's condition is _____ .

7.75. Ted Coleman required the permanent placement of a breathing tube. The procedure for the placement

of this tube is called a/an _____ .

Which Is the Correct Medical Term?

Select the correct answer and write it on the line provided.

7.76. An inflammation of the pleura that produces sharp chest pain with each breath is known as

_____ .

atelectasis   emphysema   pleurodynia   pleurisy

7.77. The substance ejected through the mouth and used for diagnostic purposes in respiratory disorders is

known as _____ _____ .

phlegm   pleural effusion   saliva   sputum

7.78. The term meaning a bluish discoloration of the skin caused by a lack of adequate oxygen is

_____ .

asphyxia   cyanosis   epistaxis   hypoxia

7.79. The medical term meaning paralysis of the vocal bands is _____ .

aphonia   dysphonia   laryngitis   laryngoplegia

7.80. The pattern of alternating periods of rapid breathing, slow breathing, and the absence of breathing is

known as _____ _____ .

anoxia   Cheyne-Stokes respiration   eupnea   tachypnea

Challenge Word Building

These terms are *not* found in this chapter; however, they are made up of the following familiar word parts. If you need help in creating the term, refer to your medical dictionary.

bronch/o	-itis
epiglott/o	-ologist
laryng/o	-plasty
pharyng/o	-plegia
pneumon/o	-rrhagia
trache/o	-rrhea
	-scopy
	-stenosis

7.81.   An abnormal discharge from the pharynx is known as _____ .

7.82.   Inflammation of the lungs is known as _____ .

7.83.   A specialist in the study of the larynx is a/an _____ .

7.84.   Bleeding from the larynx is known as _____ .

7.85.   Inflammation of both the pharynx and the larynx is known as _____ .

7.86.   Abnormal narrowing of the lumen of the trachea is known as _____ .

7.87.   The surgical repair of a bronchial defect is a/an _____ .

7.88.   Inflammation of the epiglottis is known as _____ .

7.89.   The inspection of both the trachea and bronchi through a bronchoscope is a/an _____ .

7.90.   Paralysis of the walls of the bronchi is known as _____ .

Labeling Exercises

Identify the parts of numbered items on accompanying figure

7.91. _____

7.92. _____

7.93. _____

7.94. _____ muscle

7.95. _____

7.96. _____ cavity

7.97. _____

7.98. _____

7.99. _____ lung

7.100. _____ sacs

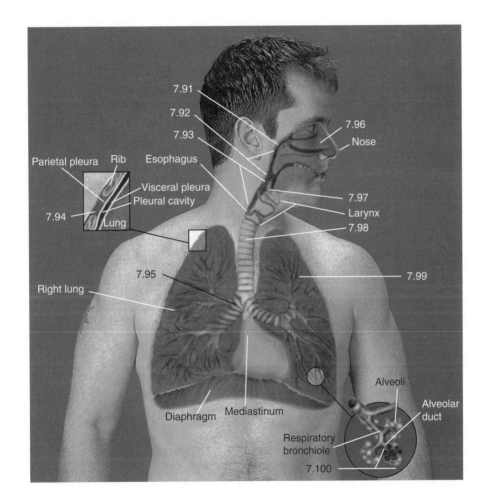

The Digestive System

Learning Exercises

Class _____   Name _____

Matching Word Parts 1
Write the correct answer in the middle column.

Definition	Correct Answer	Possible Answers
8.1. anus	_____	an/o
8.2. bile, gall	_____	chol/e
8.3. large intestine	_____	col/o
8.4. swallowing	_____	enter/o
8.5. small intestine	_____	-phagia

Matching Word Parts 2
Write the correct answer in the middle column.

Definition	Correct Answer	Possible Answers
8.6. stomach	_____	cholecyst/o
8.7. liver	_____	esophag/o
8.8. gallbladder	_____	gastr/o
8.9. esophagus	_____	hepat/o
8.10. presence of stones	_____	-lithiasis

Matching Word Parts 3
Write the correct answer in the middle column.

Definition	Correct Answer	Possible Answers
8.11. sigmoid colon	_____	-pepsia
8.12. anus and rectum	_____	-emesis
8.13. digestion	_____	proct/o
8.14. vomiting	_____	rect/o
8.15. rectum	_____	sigmoid/o

Definitions

Select the correct answer and write it on the line provided.

8.16. The visual examination of the anal canal and lower rectum is known as _____ .

    anoscopy   colonoscopy   proctoscopy   sigmoidoscopy

8.17. The term _____ means any disease of the mouth due to a fungus.

    salmonellosis   stomatomycosis   stomatoplasty   stomatorrhagia

8.18. The _____ is the last and longest portion of the small intestine.

    cecum   ileum   jejunum   pylorus

8.19. The liver removes excess _____ from the bloodstream.

    bilirubin   glucose   glycogen   lipase

8.20. The liver secretes _____ , which is stored in the gallbladder for later use.

    bile   glycogen   insulin   pepsin

8.21. The _____ _____ travels upward from the cecum to the under surface of the liver.

    ascending colon   descending colon   sigmoid colon   transverse colon

8.22. The process of the building up of body cells and substances from nutrients is known as

_____ .

    anabolism   catabolism   defecation   mastication

8.23. The receptors of taste are located on the dorsum of the _____

_____ .

    hard palate   rugae   tongue   uvula

8.24. The bone and soft tissues that surround and support the teeth are known as the

_____ .

    dentition   gingiva   occlusion   periodontium

8.25. The condition characterized by the telescoping of one part of the intestine into another is

_____ .

    borborygmus   flatus   intussusception   volvulus

Matching Structures

Write the correct answer in the middle column.

Definition	Correct Answer	Possible Answers
8.26. connects the small and large intestine	_____	cecum
8.27. S-shaped structure of the large intestine	_____	duodenum
8.28. widest division of the large intestine	_____	jejunum
8.29. middle portion of the small intestine	_____	rectum
8.30. first portion of the small intestine	_____	sigmoid colon

Which Word?

Select the correct answer and write it on the line provided.

8.31.   The medical term meaning vomiting blood is _____ .

   hematemesis   hyperemesis

8.32.   The _____ _____ virus is transmitted by the fecal oral route.

   hepatitis A   hepatitis B

8.33.   _____ is a form of food poisoning that is often fatal.

   Botulism   Bulimia

8.34.   The medical term meaning inflammation of the small intestine is _____ .

   colitis   enteritis

8.35.   The _____ hangs from the free edge of the soft palate.

   rugae   uvula

Spelling Counts

Find the misspelled word in each sentence. Then write that word, spelled correctly, on the line provided.

8.36.   An ilectomy is the surgical removal of the last portion of the small intestine. _____

8.37.   The epaglottis is a lid-like structure that prevents food and liquids from moving from the pharynx

   during swallowing. _____

8.38.   Surgical suturing of the liver is known as hepatarrhaphy. _____

8.39.   A proctoplexy is the surgical fixation of the rectum to some adjacent tissue or organ.

   _____

8.40.   The lack of adequate saliva due to the absence of or diminished secretions by the salivary glands is

   known as zerostomia. _____

Abbreviation Identification

In the space provided, write the words that each abbreviation stands for.

8.41.   **CCE**   _____

8.42.   **CRC**   _____

8.43.   **GERD**   _____

8.44.   **IBS**   _____

8.45.   **PU**   _____

Term Selection

Select the correct answer and write it on the line provided.

8.46.   The surgical removal of all or part of the stomach is a _____ .

   gastrectomy   gastritis   gastroenteritis   gastrotomy

8.47. The medical term meaning difficulty in swallowing is _____ .

      anorexia   dyspepsia   dysphagia   pyrosis

8.48. The infectious intestinal disease known as _____ _____ is caused by the one-celled parasite *Entamoeba histolytica*.

      amebic dysentery   cholera   salmonella   typhoid fever

8.49. The progressive degeneration of the liver in which scar tissue replaces normal tissue is called

_____ _____ .

      cirrhosis   hepatitis D   hepatitis E   hepatomegaly

8.50. The pigment produced by the destruction of hemoglobin in the liver is called

_____ _____ .

      bile   bilirubin   hydrochloric acid   pancreatic juice

Sentence Completion

Write the correct term on the line provided.

8.51. The excessive swallowing of air while eating or drinking is known as _____ .

8.52. The return of swallowed food to the mouth is known as _____ .

8.53. A yellow discoloration of the skin caused by greater-than-normal amounts of bilirubin in the blood is called _____ .

8.54. The _____ _____ is the ring-like muscle that controls the flow from the stomach to the small intestine.

8.55. The medical term for the solid body wastes that are expelled through the rectum is/are

_____ .

Word Surgery

Divide each term into its component word parts. Write these word parts, in sequence, on the lines provided. When necessary use a slash (/) to indicate a combining vowel. (You may not need all of the lines provided.)

8.56. An **esophagogastroduodenoscopy** is an endoscopic procedure that allows direct visualization of the upper GI tract.

_____   _____   _____   _____

8.57. A **periodontist** is a dental specialist who prevents or treats disorders of the tissues surrounding the teeth.

_____   _____   _____   _____

8.58. A **sigmoidoscopy** is the endoscopic examination of the interior of the rectum, sigmoid colon, and possibly a portion of the descending colon.

_____   _____   _____   _____

8.59. An **antiemetic** is a medication that is administered to prevent or relieve nausea and vomiting.

_____   _____   _____   _____

8.60. A **gastroduodenostomy** is the establishment of an anastomosis between the upper portion of the stomach and the duodenum.

_____   _____   _____   _____

True/False

If the statement is true, write **True** on the line. If the statement is false, write **False** on the line.

8.61. _____ Cholangitis is an acute infection of the bile duct characterized by pain in the upper right quadrant of the abdomen, fever, and jaundice.

8.62. _____ Cholangiography is an endoscopic diagnostic procedure.

8.63. _____ Acute necrotizing ulcerative gingivitis is caused by the abnormal growth of bacteria in the mouth.

8.64. _____ Bruxism means to be without natural teeth.

8.65. _____ A choledocholithotomy is an incision in the common bile duct for the removal of gallstones.

Clinical Conditions

Write the correct answer on the line provided.

8.66. James Ridgeview was diagnosed as having _____ , which is the partial or complete blockage of the small and/or large intestine.

8.67. Chang Hoon suffers from _____ . This condition is an abnormal accumulation of serous fluid in the peritoneal cavity.

8.68. Rita Martinez is a dentist. She described her patient Mr. Espinoza as being _____ , which means that he was without natural teeth.

8.69. Baby Kilgore was vomiting almost continuously. The medical term for this excessive vomiting is

_____ .

8.70. A/An _____ was performed on Mr. Schmidt to create an artificial excretory opening between his colon and body surface.

8.71. After eating, Mike Delahanty often complained about heartburn. The medical term for this condition

is _____ .

8.72. After the repeated passage of black, tarry, and foul-smelling stools, Catherine Baldwin was diagnosed

as having _____ . This condition is caused by the presence of digested blood in the stools.

8.73. Alberta Roberts was diagnosed as having an inflammation of one or more diverticula. The medical

term for this condition is _____ .

8.74. Carlotta has are blister-like sores on her lips and adjacent facial tissue. She says they are cold sores;

however, the medical term for this condition is _____ _____ .

8.75. Lisa Wilson saw her dentist because she was concerned about bad breath. Her dentist refers to this

condition as _____ .

Which Is the Correct Medical Term?

Select the correct answer and write it on the line provided.

8.76. The _____ test detects hidden blood in the stools.

anoscopy   colonoscopy   enema   Hemoccult

8.77. A/An _____ is a surgical connection between two hollow or tubular structures.

anastomosis   ostomy   stoma   sphincter

8.78. The eating disorder characterized by voluntary starvation and excessive exercising because of an intense fear of gaining weight is known as _____ _____ .

anorexia   anorexia nervosa   bulimia   bulimia nervosa

8.79. The hardened deposit that forms on the teeth and irritate the surrounding tissues is known as dental

_____ .

calculus   caries   decay   plaque

8.80. The surgical repair of the rectum is known as _____ .

anoplasty   palatoplasty   proctopexy   proctoplasty

Challenge Word Building

These terms are *not* found in this chapter; however, they are made up of the following familiar word parts. If you need help in creating the term, refer to your medical dictionary.

col/o	-algia
enter/o	-ectomy
esophag/o	-itis
gastr/o	-megaly
hepat/o	-ic
proct/o	-pexy
sigmoid/o	-rrhaphy

8.81. Surgical suturing of a stomach wound is known as _____ .

8.82. Pain in the esophagus is known as _____ .

8.83. The surgical removal of all or part of the sigmoid colon is a/an _____ .

8.84. Pain in and around the anus and rectum is known as _____ .

8.85. The surgical fixation of the stomach to correct displacement is a/an _____ .

8.86. Inflammation of the sigmoid colon is known as _____ .

8.87. The surgical removal of all or part of the esophagus and stomach is a/an _____ .

8.88. The term meaning relating to the liver and intestines is _____ .

8.89. Abnormal enlargement of the liver is known as _____ .

8.90. Inflammation of the stomach, small intestine, and large intestine is known as _____ .

Labeling Exercises

Identify the numbered items on the accompanying figure.

8.91. _____ glands

8.92. _____

8.93. _____

8.94. _____

8.95. _____

8.96. _____

8.97. _____ intestine

8.98. vermiform _____

8.99. _____ intestine

8.100. _____ and anus

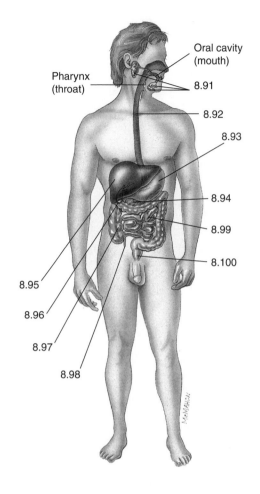

CHAPTER 9

The Urinary System

Learning Exercises

Class _____   Name _____

Matching Word Parts 1
Write the correct answer in the middle column.

Definition	Correct Answer	Possible Answers
9.1. bladder	_____	-cele
9.2. glomerulus	_____	cyst/o
9.3. hernia, tumor, cyst	_____	glomerul/o
9.4. kidney	_____	lith/o
9.5. stone, calculus	_____	nephr/o

Matching Word Parts 2
Write the correct answer in the middle column.

Definition	Correct Answer	Possible Answers
9.6. drooping down	_____	-tripsy
9.7. renal pelvis	_____	pyel/o
9.8. setting free, separation	_____	-ptosis
9.9. surgical fixation	_____	-pexy
9.10. to crush	_____	-lysis

Matching Word Parts 3
Write the correct answer in the middle column.

Definition	Correct Answer	Possible Answers
9.11. complete, through	_____	-uria
9.12. enlargement, stretching	_____	urethr/o
9.13. ureter	_____	ureter/o
9.14. urethra	_____	-ectasis
9.15. urination, urine	_____	dia-

Definitions

Select the correct answer and write it on the line provided.

9.16. Urine is carried from the kidneys to the urinary bladder by the _____ .

    glomeruli   nephrons   urethras   ureters

9.17. A stone in the urinary bladder is known as a _____ .

    cholelith   cystolith   nephrolith   ureterolith

9.18. The increased output of urine is known as _____ .

    anuria   diuresis   dysuria   oliguria

9.19. Before entering the ureters, urine collects in the _____ _____ .

    glomeruli   renal cortex   renal pelvis   urinary bladder

9.20. Urine leaves the bladder through the _____ .

    prostate   trigone   ureter   urethra

9.21. Urine gets its normal yellow-amber or straw color from the pigment known as _____ .

    albumin   bilirubin   hemoglobin   urochrome

9.22. In the male, the _____ _____ carries both urine and semen.

    prostate gland   renal pelvis   ureter   urethra

9.23. A specialist who treats the genitourinary system of males is a/an _____ .

    gynecologist   nephrologist   neurologist   urologist

9.24. In _____ , the urethral opening is on one side of the penis.

    epispadias   hyperspadias   hypospadias   paraspadias

9.25. The term _____ describes treatment in which a body part is removed or its function is destroyed. This type of procedure is frequently used to treat prostate cancer.

    ablation   adhesion   lithotomy   meatotomy

Matching Structures

Write the correct answer in the middle column.

Definition	Correct Answer	Possible Answers
9.26. the opening through which urine leaves the body	_____	urethral meatus
9.27. the portion of a nephron that is active in filtering urine	_____	urethra
9.28. the outer layer of the kidney	_____	ureters
9.29. the tube from the bladder to the outside of the body	_____	renal cortex
9.30. the tubes that carry urine from the kidney to the bladder	_____	glomerulus

Which Word?

Select the correct answer and write it on the line provided.

9.31. A surgical incision into the renal pelvis is _____ .

    pyelotomy   pyeloplasty

9.32. The discharge of blood from the ureter is _____ .

    ureterorrhagia   urethrorrhagia

9.33. The term meaning excessive urination is _____ .

    incontinence   polyuria

9.34. The term meaning inflammation of the bladder is _____ .

    cystitis   pyelitis

9.35. The major waste product of protein metabolism is _____ .

    urea   urine

Spelling Counts

Find the misspelled word in each sentence. Then write that word, spelled correctly, on the line provided.

9.36. A Williams tumor is a malignant tumor of the kidney that occurs in children.

    _____

9.37. Being unable to control excretory functions is known as incontinance. _____

9.38. The process of withdrawing urine from the bladder is known as catherozation.

    _____

9.39. Kagel exercises are a series of pelvic muscle exercises used to strengthen the muscles of the pelvic floor to control urinary stress incontinence. _____

9.40. A vescikovaginal fistula is an abnormal opening between the bladder and vagina

    _____ .

Abbreviation Identification

In the space provided, write the words that each abbreviation stands for.

9.41. **BPH** _____

9.42. **ESRD** _____

9.43. **ESWL** _____

9.44. **IVP** _____

9.45. **OAB** _____

Term Selection

Select the correct answer and write it on the line provided.

9.46. The absence of urine formation by the kidneys is known as _____ .

    anuria   nocturia   oliguria   polyuria

9.47. The surgical suturing of the bladder is known as _____ .

    cystorrhaphy   cystorrhagia   cystorrhexis   nephrorrhaphy

9.48. The term meaning the freeing of a kidney from adhesions is _____ .

    nephrolithiasis   nephrolysis   nephropyosis   pyelitis

9.49. The term meaning scanty urination is _____ .

| diuresis | dysuria | enuresis | oliguria |

9.50. The process of artificially filtering waste products from the patient's blood is known as _____ .

| diuresis | hemodialysis | homeostasis | hydroureter |

Sentence Completion
Write the correct term on the line provided.

9.51. An inflammation of the urinary bladder that is localized in the region of the trigone is known as

_____ .

9.52. The condition of having a stone lodged in a ureter is known as _____ .

9.53. The placement of a catheter into the bladder through a small incision made through the abdominal

wall just above the pubic bone is known as _____ _____ .

9.54. The surgical fixation of the bladder to the abdominal wall is a/an _____ .

9.55. A/An _____ _____ of the prostate (TURP) is the removal of all or part of the prostate through the urethra.

Word Surgery
Divide each term into its component word parts. Write these word parts, in sequence, on the lines provided. When necessary use a back slash (/) to indicate a combining vowel. (You may not need all of the lines provided.)

9.56. **Hyperproteinuria** is abnormally high concentrations of protein in the urine.

_____ _____ _____ _____

9.57. **Hydronephrosis** is the dilation of the renal pelvis of one or both kidneys.

_____ _____ _____ _____

9.58. Voiding **cystourethrography** is a diagnostic procedure in which a fluoroscope is used to examine the flow of urine from the bladder and through the urethra.

_____ _____ _____ _____

9.59. A **nephrolithotomy** is the surgical removal of a kidney stone through an incision in the kidney.

_____ _____ _____ _____

9.60. **Lithotripsy** means to crush a stone.

_____ _____ _____ _____

True/False
If the statement is true, write **True** on the line. If the statement is false, write **False** on the line.

9.61. _____ Stress incontinence is the inability to control the voiding of urine under physical stress such as running, sneezing, laughing, or coughing.

9.62. _____ Prostatism is a malignancy of the prostate gland.

9.63. _____ Urethrorrhea is bleeding from the urethra.

9.64. _____ Renal colic is an acute pain in the kidney area that is caused by blockage during the passage of a kidney stone.

9.65. _____ Acute renal failure has sudden onset and is characterized by uremia.

Clinical Conditions

Write the correct answer on the line provided.

9.66. Mr. Baldridge suffers from excessive urination during the night. The medical term for this is

_____ .

9.67. Rosita LaPinta inherited _____ kidney disease. These cysts slowly reduce the kidney function, and this eventually leads to kidney failure.

9.68. Doris Volk has a chronic bladder condition involving inflammation within the wall of the bladder. This is known as _____ _____ .

9.69. John Danielson has an enlarged prostate gland. This caused narrowing of the urethra, which is known as _____ .

9.70. Norman Smith was born with the opening of the urethra on the upper surface of the penis. This is known as _____ .

9.71. Henry Wong's kidneys failed. He is being treated with _____ _____ , which involves the removal of waste from his blood through a fluid exchange in the abdominal cavity.

9.72. Roberta Gridley is scheduled for surgical repair of damage to the ureter. This procedure is a/an

_____ .

9.73. When Larry's _____ _____ blood test showed a very high PSA level, his physician was concerned about the possibility of prostate cancer.

9.74. Dr. Morita's patient was diagnosed as having _____ , which is also known as Bright's disease. This is a type of kidney disease caused by inflammation of the glomeruli that causes red blood cells and proteins to leak into the urine.

9.75. Mrs. Franklin describes her condition as a floating kidney. The medical term for this condition, in which there is a downward displacement of the kidney, is _____ .

Which Is the Correct Medical Term?

Select the correct answer and write it on the line provided.

9.76. Acute renal failure has sudden onset and is characterized by _____ . This condition can be caused by many factors, including a sudden drop in blood volume or blood pressure due to injury or surgery.

anuria   dysuria   enuresis   uremia

9.77. The term _____ _____ is urinary incontinence during sleep. It is also known as bed-wetting.

nocturnal enuresis   overactive bladder   stress incontinence   urinary incontinence

9.78. The term meaning the distention of the ureter is _____ .

ureteritis   ureterectasis   ureterolith   urethrostenosis

9.79. The presence of abnormally *low* concentrations of protein in the blood is known as

_____ .

hypertrophy   hyperproteinuria   hypocalcemia   hypoproteinemia

9.80. A specialist in diagnosing and treating diseases and disorders of the kidneys is a/an

_____ .

gynecologist   nephrologist   proctologist   urologist

Challenge Word Building

These terms are *not* found in this chapter; however, they are made up of the following familiar word parts. If you need help in creating the term, refer to your medical dictionary.

cyst/o	-cele
nephr/o	-itis
pyel/o	-lysis
ureter/o	-malacia
urethr/o	-ostomy
	-otomy
	-plasty
	-ptosis
	-rrhexis
	-sclerosis

9.81. The creation of an artificial opening between the urinary bladder and the exterior of the body is a/an

_____ .

9.82. A surgical incision into the kidney is a/an _____ .

9.83. Abnormal hardening of the kidney is known as _____ .

9.84. Prolapse of the bladder into the urethra is known as _____ .

9.85. A hernia in the urethral wall is a/an _____ .

9.86. The procedure to separate adhesions around a ureter is a/an _____ .

9.87. Abnormal softening of the kidney is known as _____ .

9.88. Inflammation of the renal pelvis and kidney is known as _____ .

9.89. Rupture of the urinary bladder is known as _____ .

9.90. The surgical repair of the bladder is a/an _____ .

Labeling Exercises

Identify the numbered items on the accompanying figure.

9.91. _____ gland

9.92. exterior view of the right

_____

9.93. inferior _____

_____

9.94. _____

9.95. renal _____

9.96. renal _____

9.97. abdominal _____

9.98. right and left _____

9.99. urinary _____

9.100. urethral _____

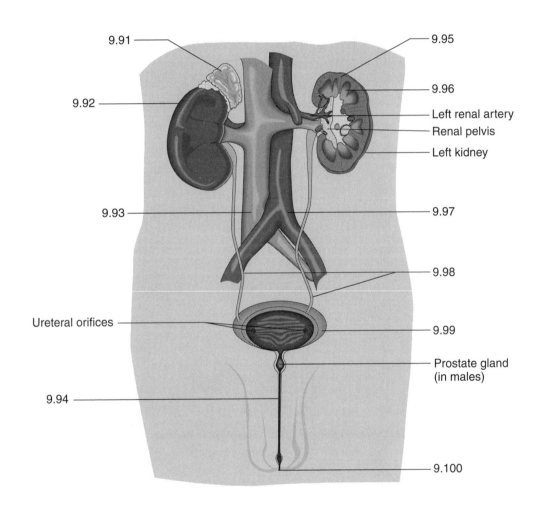

The Nervous System

Learning Exercises

Class _____   Name _____

Matching Word Parts 1
Write the correct answer in the middle column.

Definition	Correct Answer	Possible Answers
10.1. feeling	_____	psych/o
10.2. brain	_____	encephal/o
10.3. bruise	_____	contus/o
10.4. mind	_____	concuss/o
10.5. shaken together	_____	esthet/o

Matching Word Parts 2
Write the correct answer in the middle column.

Definition	Correct Answer	Possible Answers
10.6. brain covering	_____	-esthesia
10.7. process of recording an image	_____	-graphy
10.8. sensation, feeling	_____	klept/o
10.9. spinal cord	_____	mening/o
10.10. to steal	_____	myel/o

Matching Word Parts 3
Write the correct answer in the middle column.

Definition	Correct Answer	Possible Answers
10.11. abnormal fear	_____	-tropic
10.12. burning sensation	_____	-phobia
10.13. madness	_____	neur/o
10.14. nerve, nerves	_____	-mania
10.15. having an affinity for	_____	caus/o

Definitions

Select the correct answer and write it on the line provided.

10.16. The space between two neurons or between a neuron and a receptor is known as a

_____ .

    dendrite   ganglion   plexus   synapse

10.17. The white protective covering over some nerve cells is the _____

_____ .

    myelin sheath   neuroglia   neurotransmitter   pia mater

10.18. The _____ are the root-like structures of a nerve that receive impulses and conduct them to the cell body.

    axons   dendrites   ganglions   neurotransmitters

10.19. The _____ _____ is the layer of the meninges that is located nearest the brain and spinal cord.

    arachnoid membrane   dura mater   meninx   pia mater

10.20. Seven vital body functions are controlled by the _____ .

    cerebral cortex   cerebellum   hypothalamus   thalamus

10.21. The _____ nervous system is the division of the autonomic nervous system that is concerned with body functions.

    afferent   parasympathetic   peripheral   sympathetic

10.22. A _____ is a network of intersecting nerves.

    ganglion   plexus   synapse   tract

10.23. Cranial nerves are part of the _____ nervous system.

    autonomic   central   cranial   peripheral

10.24. The _____ relays sensory stimuli from the spinal cord and midbrain to the cerebral cortex.

    cerebellum   hypothalamus   medulla   thalamus

10.25. The _____ neurons carry impulses away from the brain and spinal cord.

    afferent   associative   efferent   sensory

Matching Structures

Write the correct answer in the middle column.

Definition	Correct Answer	Possible Answers
10.26. connects the brain and spinal cord	_____	medulla
10.27. controls vital body functions	_____	hypothalamus
10.28. coordinates muscular activity	_____	cerebrum
10.29. most protected brain part	_____	cerebellum
10.30. uppermost layer of the brain	_____	brainstem

Which Word?

Select the correct answer and write it on the line provided.

10.31. A physician who specializes in administering anesthetic agents is an _____ .

anesthetist anesthesiologist

10.32. A _____ is a profound state of unconsciousness marked by the absence of spontaneous eye movements, no response to painful stimuli, and the lack of speech.

coma stupor

10.33. An _____ drug is also known as a tranquilizer.

antipsychotic anxiolytic

10.34. A/An _____ is a sense perception that has no basis in external stimulation.

delusion hallucination

10.35. An excessive fear of heights is _____ .

acrophobia agoraphobia

Spelling Counts

Find the misspelled word in each sentence. Then write that word, spelled correctly, on the line provided.

10.36. A miagraine headache is characterized by throbbing pain on one side of the head.

_____

10.37. Altzheimer's disease is a group disorders involving the parts of the brain that control thought, memory, and language. _____

10.38. An anesthethic is medication that is administered to block the normal sensation of pain.

_____

10.39. Epalepsy is a chronic neurological condition characterized by recurrent episodes of seizures of varying severity. _____

10.40. Schiatica is a nerve inflammation that may result in pain through the thigh and leg.

_____

Abbreviation Identification

In the space provided, write the words that each abbreviation stands for.

10.41. **CP** _____

10.42. **CVA** _____

10.43. **OCD** _____

10.44. **PTSD** _____

10.45. **TIA** _____

Term Selection

Select the correct answer and write it on the line provided.

10.46. The acute condition caused by a high fever that is characterized by confusion, disorientation, disordered thinking, agitation, and hallucinations is known as _____ .

      delirium   dementia   lethargy   stupor

10.47. The term meaning inflammation of the spinal cord is _____ . This term also means inflammation of bone marrow.

      encephalitis   myelitis   myelosis   radiculitis

10.48. The medical term meaning an abnormal fear of being in narrow or enclosed spaces is

      _____ .

      acrophobia   claustrophobia   kleptomania   pyromania

10.49. The condition known as _____ _____ is characterized by severe lightning-like pain due to an inflammation of the fifth cranial nerve.

      Bell's palsy   Guillain-Barré syndrome   Lou Gehrig's disease   trigeminal neuralgia

10.50. The medical term for the condition also known as a developmental reading disorder is

      _____ _____ .

      autism   dissociative disorder   dyslexia   mental retardation

Sentence Completion

Write the correct term on the line provided.

10.51. A _____ _____ is the bruising of brain tissue as a result of a head injury.

10.52. The mental conditions characterized by excessive, irrational dread of everyday situations or fear that is out of proportion to the real danger in a situation are known as _____ _____ .

10.53. The disorder characterized by repeated, deliberate fire setting is known as _____ .

10.54. A/An _____ disorder is a condition in which an individual acts as if he or she has a physical or mental illness when he or she is not really sick.

10.55. A/An _____ drug is administered to treat severe mental disorders including schizophrenia and mania.

Word Surgery

Divide each term into its component word parts. Write these word parts, in sequence, on the lines provided. When necessary use a slash (/) to indicate a combining vowel. (You may not need all of the lines provided.)

10.56. An **anesthetic** is the medication used to induce the loss of normal sensation, especially sensitivity to pain.

      _____   _____   _____   _____

10.57. **Somnambulism** is commonly known as sleepwalking.

      _____   _____   _____   _____

10.58. **Electroencephalography** is the process of recording the electrical activity of the brain through the use of electrodes attached to the scalp.

_____   _____   _____   _____

10.59. **Echoencephalography** is the use of ultrasound imaging to diagnose a shift in the midline structures of the brain.

_____   _____   _____   _____

10.60. **Poliomyelitis** is a viral infection of the gray matter of the spinal cord that may result in paralysis.

_____   _____   _____   _____

True/False

If the statement is true, write **True** on the line. If the statement is false, write **False** on the line.

10.61. _____ A hemorrhagic stroke occurs when a blood vessel in the brain leaks.

10.62. _____ Arachnophobia is an excessive fear of spiders.

10.63. _____ A sedative is administered to prevent the seizures associated with epilepsy.

10.64. _____ A patient in a persistent vegetative state sleeps through the night and is awake during the day.

10.65. _____ A psychotropic drug acts primarily on the central nervous system where it produces temporary changes affecting the mind, emotions, and behavior.

Clinical Conditions

Write the correct answer on the line provided.

10.66. Harvey Ikeman has mood shifts from highs to severe lows that affect his mood, energy, and ability to function. Harvey's doctor describes this condition as a/an _____ disorder.

10.67. In the auto accident, Anthony DeNicola hit his head on the windshield. The paramedics were concerned that this jarring of the brain had caused a/an _____ .

10.68. Georgia Houghton suffered a _____ _____ attack (TIA), and her doctors were concerned that this was a warning of an impending stroke.

10.69. To control her patient's tremors caused by Parkinson's disease, Dr. Wang performed a/an _____ . This is a surgical incision into the thalamus.

10.70. Mary Beth Cawthorn was diagnosed as having _____ _____ (MS). This autoimmune disease is characterized by patches of demyelinated nerve fibers.

10.71. After several months of being unable to sleep well, Wayne Ladner visited his doctor about this problem. His doctor recorded this condition as being _____ .

10.72. After her stroke, Rosita Valladares was unable to understand written or spoken words. This condition is known as _____ .

10.73. Jill Beck said she fainted. The medical term for this brief loss of consciousness caused by a lack of oxygen in the brain is _____ .

10.74. The Baily baby was born with _____ . This condition is an abnormally increased amount of cerebrospinal fluid within the brain.

10.75. The MRI indicated that Mrs. Hoshi had a collection of blood trapped in the tissues of her brain. This condition, which was caused by a head injury, is called a cranial _____ .

Which Is the Correct Medical Term?

Select the correct answer and write it on the line provided.

10.76. Persistent severe burning pain that usually follows an injury to a sensory nerve is known as

_____ .

causalgia   hyperesthesia   hypoesthesia   paresthesia

10.77. The classification of drug that depresses the central nervous system and usually produces sleep is

known as a/an _____ .

anesthetic   barbiturate   hypnotic   sedative

10.78. A/An _____ disorder is characterized by serious temporary or ongoing changes in function, such as paralysis or blindness, which are triggered by psychological factors rather than by any physical cause.

anxiety   conversion   factitious   panic

10.79. During childbirth, _____ anesthesia is administered to numb the nerves from the uterus and birth passage without stopping labor.

epidural   local   regional   topical

10.80. The condition known as _____ _____

_____ (ALS) is a rapidly progressive neurological disease that attacks the nerve cells responsible for controlling voluntary muscles.

amyotrophic lateral sclerosis   cerebral palsy   epilepsy   multiple sclerosis

Challenge Word Building

These terms are *not* found in this chapter; however, they are made up of the following familiar word parts. If you need help in creating the term, refer to your medical dictionary.

poly-	encephal/o	-algia
	mening/o	-itis
	myel/o	-malacia
	neur/o	-oma
		-pathy

10.81. Based on word parts, the term meaning any disease or disorders of a nerve or nerves is

_____ .

10.82. Abnormal softening of the meninges is known as _____ .

10.83. A benign neoplasm made up of nerve tissue is a/an _____ .

10.84. Based on word parts, the term meaning any degenerative disease of the brain is

_____ .

10.85. An inflammation affecting many nerves is known as _____ .

10.86. Abnormal softening of nerve tissue is known as _____ .

10.87. Inflammation of the meninges and the brain is known as _____ .

10.88. Based on word parts, the term meaning any pathological condition of the spinal cord is

_____ .

10.89. Abnormal softening of the brain is known as _____ .

10.90. Inflammation of the meninges, brain, and spinal cord is known as _____ .

Labeling Exercises
Identify the numbered items on the accompanying figures.

10.91. _____ cortex   10.96. _____

10.92. _____ lobe   10.97. _____

10.93. _____ lobe   10.98. _____

10.94. _____ lobe   10.99. _____ cord

10.95. _____ lobe   10.100. _____

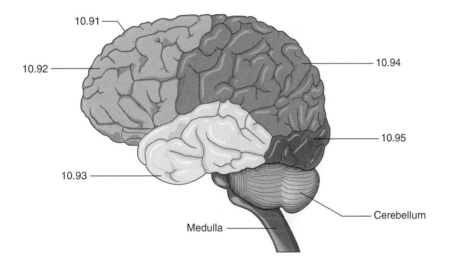

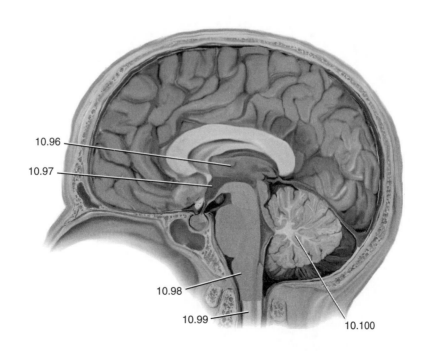

CHAPTER 11

Special Senses: The Eyes and Ears

Learning Exercises

Class _____   Name _____

Matching Word Parts 1
Write the correct answer in the middle column.

Definition	Correct Answer	Possible Answers
11.1. cornea, hard	_____	opt/o
11.2. eyelid	_____	-metry
11.3. eyes, vision	_____	kerat/o
11.4. hearing	_____	-cusis
11.5. to measure	_____	blephar/o

Matching Word Parts 2
Write the correct answer in the middle column.

Definition	Correct Answer	Possible Answers
11.6. eardrum	_____	presby/o
11.7. eye, vision	_____	-opia
11.8. iris of the eye	_____	ophthalm/o
11.9. old age	_____	myring/o
11.10. vision condition	_____	irid/o

Matching Word Parts 3
Write the correct answer in the middle column.

Definition	Correct Answer	Possible Answers
11.11. ear	_____	tympan/o
11.12. eardrum	_____	trop/o
11.13. hard, white of eye	_____	scler/o
11.14. retina	_____	retin/o
11.15. turn	_____	ot/o

Definitions
Select the correct answer and write it on the line provided.

11.16. The _____ is the structure that maintains the shape of the eye and protects the delicate inner tissues.

    choroid   conjunctiva   cornea   sclera

11.17. The _____ _____ is the snail-shaped, fluid-filled structure that forms the inner ear.

    cochlea   eustachian tube   organ of Corti   semicircular canal

11.18. The _____ _____ is also known as the blind spot of the eye.

    fovea centralis   macula   optic disk   optic nerve

11.19. The _____ _____ lies between the outer ear and the middle ear.

    mastoid cells   oval window   pinna   tympanic membrane

11.20. The _____ _____ separates the middle ear from the inner ear.

    eustachian tube   inner canthus   oval window   tympanic membrane

11.21. The auditory ossicle, which is also known as the anvil, is the _____ .

    incus   labyrinth   malleus   stapes

11.22. The term meaning lessening of the accommodation of the lens that occurs normally with aging is _____ .

    ametropia   amblyopia   presbyopia   presbycusis

11.23. Laser _____ is used to repair a detached retina.

    keratoplasty   photocoagulation   retinopexy   trabeculoplasty

11.24. The turning inward of the edge of the eyelid is known as _____ .

    ectropion   emmetropia   entropion   esotropia

11.25. Acute _____ otitis media is a buildup of pus within the middle ear.

    effusive   inflammatory   purulent   serous

Matching Conditions
Write the correct answer in the middle column.

Definition	Correct Answer	Possible Answers
11.26. cross-eyes	_____	strabismus
11.27. double vision	_____	myopia
11.28. farsightedness	_____	hyperopia
11.29. nearsightedness	_____	esotropia
11.30. squint	_____	diplopia

Which Word?
Select the correct answer and write it on the line provided.

11.31. A _____ is the unit of measurement of a lens' refractive power.

     decibel   diopter

11.32. The term meaning bleeding from the ears is _____ .

     otorrhagia   otorrhea

11.33. A _____ is the surgical incision of the eardrum to create an opening for the placement of tympanostomy tubes.

     myringotomy   tympanoplasty

11.34. A visual field test to determine losses in peripheral vision is used to diagnose _____ .

     cataracts   glaucoma

11.35. A _____ hearing test that involves both ears.

     binaural   binocular

Spelling Counts
Find the misspelled word in each sentence. Then write that word, spelled correctly, on the line provided.

11.36. The euctachian tubes lead from the middle ear to the nasal cavity and the throat.

     _____

11.37. Cerunem, also known as earwax, is secreted by glands that line the external auditory canal.

     _____

11.38. Astegmatism is a condition in which the eye does not focus properly because of uneven curvatures of the cornea. _____

11.39. A laberinthotomy is a surgical incision between two of the fluid chambers of the labyrinth to allow the pressure to equalize. _____

11.40. A Snellan chart is used to measure visual acuity. _____

Abbreviation Identification

In the space provided, write the words that each abbreviation stands for.

11.41. **AS** _____

11.42. **IOL** _____

11.43. **OD** _____

11.44. **IOP** _____

11.45. **MD** _____

Term Selection

Select the correct answer and write it on the line provided.

11.46. A radial keratotomy is performed to treat _____ .

    cataracts   hyperopia   myopia   strabismus

11.47. The condition in which the pupils are unequal in size is known as _____
_____ .

    anisocoria   choked disk   macular degeneration   synechia

11.48. A _____ is performed in preparation for the placement of a cochlear implant.

    keratoplasty   labyrinthectomy   mastoidectomy   myringoplasty

11.49. The condition also known as a stye is _____ _____ .

    blepharoptosis   chalazion   hordeolum   subconjunctival hemorrhage

11.50. The medical term for the condition commonly known as swimmer's ear is _____ .

    otalgia   otitis   otomycosis   otopyorrhea

Sentence Completion

Write the correct term on the line provided.

11.51. The ability of the lens to bend light rays so they focus on the retina is known as

_____ .

11.52. A sense of whirling, dizziness, and the loss of balance is called _____ .

11.53. A/An _____ is a specialist in measuring the accuracy of vision.

11.54. An inflammation of the cornea that can be due to many causes, including bacterial, viral, or fungal

infections, is known as _____ .

11.55. The medical term meaning color blindness is _____ .

Word Surgery

Divide each term into its component word parts. Write these word parts, in sequence, on the lines provided.
When necessary use a slash (/) to indicate a combining vowel. (You may not need all of the lines provided.)

11.56. **Ophthalmoscopy** is the visual examination of the fundus of the eye.

_____   _____   _____   _____

11.57. **Emmetropia** is the normal relationship between the refractive power of the eye and the shape of the
eye that enables light rays to focus correctly on the retina.

_____   _____   _____   _____   _____

11.58. **Otopyorrhea** is the flow of pus from the ear.

_____   _____   _____   _____

11.59. **Presbycusis** is a gradual loss of sensorineural hearing that occurs as the body ages.

_____   _____   _____   _____

11.60. **Xerophthalmia** is drying of eye surfaces, including the conjunctiva, that is often associated with aging.

_____   _____   _____   _____

True/False

If the statement is true, write **True** on the line. If the statement is false, write **False** on the line.

11.61. _____ Rods in the retina are the receptors for color.

11.62. _____ Aqueous fluid is drained through the canal of Schlemm.

11.63. _____ Visual field testing is performed to determine the presence of cataracts.

11.64. _____ Dacryoadenitis is an inflammation of the lacrimal gland that can be caused by a bacterial, viral, or fungal infection.

11.65. _____ Tarsorrhaphy is the suturing together of the upper and lower eyelids.

Clinical Conditions

Write the correct answer on the line provided.

11.66. Following a boxing match, Jack Lawson required _____ to repair the injured pinna of his ear.

11.67. During his scuba diving expedition, Jose Ortega suffered from pressure-related ear discomfort. The medical term for this condition is _____ .

11.68. Margo Spencer was diagnosed with closed-angle glaucoma affecting her left eye. She is scheduled to have a/an _____ performed to treat this condition.

11.69. Edward Cooke was diagnosed as having _____ . This condition is characterized by blindness in one-half of the visual field.

11.70. While gathering branches after the storm, Vern Passman scratched the cornea of his eye. To diagnose the damage, his ophthalmologist performed _____ staining, which caused the corneal abrasions to appear bright green.

11.71. Ted Milligan was treated for an allergic reaction to being stung by a wasp. His reaction was swelling around his eyes, and this is known as _____ edema.

11.72. Adrienne Jacobus is unable to drive at night because she suffers from night blindness. The medical term for this condition is _____ .

11.73. James Escobar complained of a ringing sound in his ears. His physician refers to this condition as

_____ .

11.74. Although it is a benign growth, the _____ on Ingrid's eye required treatment because it had grown large enough to distort her vision.

11.75. Susie Harris was diagnosed as having _____ . Her mother referred to this condition as pinkeye.

Which Is the Correct Medical Term?

Select the correct answer and write it on the line provided.

11.76. Commonly known as choked disk, _____ is swelling and inflammation of the optic nerve at the point of entrance into the eye through the optic disk.

    eustachitis   papilledema   tinnitus   xerophthalmia

11.77. An adhesion that binds the iris to an adjacent structure such as the lens or cornea is known as

_____ .

    blepharoptosis   convergence   scleritis   synechia

11.78. The term _____ describes any error of refraction in which images do not focus properly on the retina.

    ametropia   diplopia   esotropia   hemianopia

11.79. A _____ is a localized swelling inside the eyelid resulting from obstruction of one of the sebaceous glands.

    chalazion   hordeolum   papilledema   pterygium

11.80. The term _____ _____ describes an accumulation of earwax in the auditory canal.

    canthus   impacted cerumen   otitis externa   pseudophakia

Challenge Word Building

These terms are *not* found in this chapter; however, they are made up of the following familiar word parts. If you need help in creating the term, refer to your medical dictionary.

blephar/o	-algia
irid/o	-ectomy
lacrim/o	-edema
ophthalm/o	-itis
labyrinth/o	-ology
retin/o	-otomy
	-pathy

11.81. Pain felt in the iris is known as _____ .

11.82. Inflammation of the eyelid is known as _____ .

11.83. An incision into the iris is a/an _____ .

11.84. The term _____ means any disease of the retina.

11.85. The medical specialty concerned with the eye, its diseases, and refractive errors is known as

_____ .

11.86. Swelling of the eyelid is known as _____ .

11.87. A surgical incision into the lacrimal duct is a/an _____ .

11.88. The surgical removal of the labyrinth of the inner ear is a/an _____ .

11.89. The term meaning any disease of the iris is _____ .

11.90. Inflammation of the retina is known as _____ .

Labeling Exercises

Identify the numbered items on the accompanying figures.

11.91. _____

11.92. anterior _____

11.93. crystalline _____

11.94. _____

11.95. _____ centralis

11.96. _____ or pinna

11.97. external _____ canal

11.98. _____ membrane

11.99. _____ tube

11.100. _____

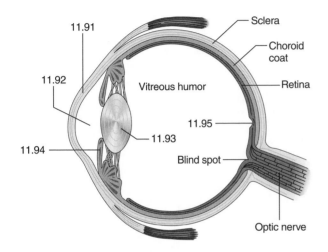

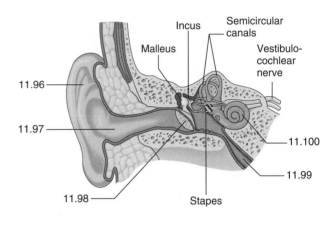

CHAPTER 12

Skin: The Integumentary System

Learning Exercises

Class _____   Name _____

Matching Word Parts 1
Write the correct answer in the middle column.

Definition	Correct Answer	Possible Answers
12.1. life	_____	urtic/o
12.2. rash	_____	rhytid/o
12.3. red	_____	hidr/o
12.4. sweat	_____	erythr/o
12.5. wrinkle	_____	bi/o

Matching Word Parts 2
Write the correct answer in the middle column.

Definition	Correct Answer	Possible Answers
12.6. black, dark	_____	pedicul/o
12.7. fat, lipid	_____	melan/o
12.8. horny, hard	_____	lip/o
12.9. lice	_____	kerat/o
12.10. skin	_____	dermat/o

Matching Word Parts 3

Write the correct answer in the middle column.

Definition	Correct Answer	Possible Answers
12.11. dry	_____	xer/o
12.12. fungus	_____	seb/o
12.13. hairy	_____	onych/o
12.14. nail	_____	myc/o
12.15. sebum	_____	hirsut/o

Definitions

Select the correct answer and write it on the line provided.

12.16. An acute, rapidly spreading infection within the connective tissues is known as

_____ .

    abscess   cellulitis   fissure   ulcer

12.17. Atypical moles that can develop into skin cancer are known as _____

_____ .

    dysplastic nevi   lipomas   malignant keratoses   papillomas

12.18. The autoimmune disorder in which there are well-defined bald areas is known as

_____ _____ .

    alopecia areata   alopecia capitis   alopecia universalis   psoriasis

12.19. A/An _____ is a swelling of clotted blood trapped in the tissues.

    abscess   contusion   hematoma   petechiae

12.20. The term _____ means profuse sweating.

    anhidrosis   diaphoresis   hidrosis   miliaria

12.21. A normal scar resulting from the healing of a wound is called a _____ .

    cicatrix   keloid   keratosis   papilloma

12.22. A large blister that is usually more than 0.5 cm in diameter is known as a/an _____ .

    abscess   bulla   pustule   vesicle

12.23. The removal of dirt, foreign objects, damaged tissue, and cellular debris from a wound is called

_____ .

    cauterization   curettage   debridement   dermabrasion

12.24. A _____-_____ burn has blisters plus damage only to the epidermis and dermis.

    first-degree   fourth-degree   second-degree   third-degree

12.25. Commonly known as warts, _____ are small, hard, skin lesions caused by the human papilloma virus.

    nevi   petechiae   scabies   verrucae

Matching Structures

Write the correct answer in the middle column.

Definition	Correct Answer	Possible Answers
12.26. fibrous protein found in hair, nails, and skin	_____	unguis
12.27. fingernails and toenails	_____	sebaceous glands
12.28. glands secreting sebum	_____	mammary glands
12.29. milk-producing sebaceous glands	_____	keratin
12.30. the layer of skin below the epidermis	_____	dermis

Which Word?

Select the correct answer and write it on the line provided.

12.31. The medical term for the condition commonly known as an ingrown toenail is

_____ .

onychomycosis   onychocryptosis

12.32. The bacterial skin infection characterized by isolated pustules that become crusted and rupture

is known as _____ . This highly contagious condition commonly occurs in

children.

impetigo   xeroderma

12.33. A torn or jagged wound or an accidental cut wound is known as a _____ .

laceration   lesion

12.34. The lesions of _____ _____ carcinoma tend to bleed easily.

basal cell   squamous cell

12.35. Group A strep, also known as flesh-eating bacteria, causes _____

_____ .

lupus erythematosus   necrotizing fasciitis

Spelling Counts

Find the misspelled word in each sentence. Then write that word, spelled correctly, on the line provided.

12.36. Soriasis is a chronic disease of the skin characterized by itching and by red papules covered with silvery

scales. _____

12.37. Exema is an inflammatory skin disease with erythema, papules, and scabs. _____

12.38. An absess is a localized collection of pus. _____

12.39. Onyochia is an inflammation of the nail bed that usually results in the loss of the nail.

_____

12.40. Skleroderma is an autoimmune disorder in which the connective tissues become thickened and

hardened, causing the skin to become hard and swollen. _____

Abbreviation Identification

In the space provided, write the words that each abbreviation stands for.

12.41. **BCC, BCCA** _____

12.42. **I & D** _____

12.43. **LE** _____

12.44. **MM, mm** _____

12.45. **SCC** _____

Term Selection

Select the correct answer and write it on the line provided.

12.46. A _____ is small, knot-like swelling of granulation tissue in the epidermis.

cicatrix   granuloma   keratosis   petechiae

12.47. An infestation of body lice is known as _____ _____ .

pediculosis capitis   pediculosis corporis   pediculosis pubis   scabies

12.48. The term _____ is used to describe any redness of the skin due to dilated capillaries.

dermatitis   ecchymosis   erythema   urticaria

12.49. Flakes or dry patches made up of excess dead epidermal cells are a known as

_____ .

bullae   macules   plaques   scales

12.50. A cluster of connected boils is known as a/an _____ .

acne vulgaris   carbuncle   comedo   furuncle

Sentence Completion

Write the correct term on the line provided.

12.51. The term meaning producing or containing pus is _____ .

12.52. The term meaning a fungal infection of the nail is _____ .

12.53. Tissue death followed by bacterial invasion and putrefaction is known as _____ .

12.54. Any condition of unusual deposits of black pigment in different parts of the body is known as

_____ .

12.55. Commonly known as hives, _____ are itchy welts caused by an allergic reaction.

Word Surgery

Divide each term into its component word parts. Write these word parts, in sequence, on the lines provided. When necessary use a slash (/) to indicate a combining vowel. (You may not need all of the lines provided.)

12.56. A **rhytidectomy** is the surgical removal of excess skin for the elimination of wrinkles.

_____   _____   _____   _____

12.57. **Onychomycosis** is a fungal infection of the nail.

_____   _____   _____   _____

12.58. **Folliculitis** is an inflammation of the hair follicles that is especially common on the limbs and in the beard area of men.

_____   _____   _____   _____

12.59. **Pruritus**, which is commonly known as itching, is associated with most forms of dermatitis.

_____   _____   _____   _____

12.60. **Ichthyosis** is a group of hereditary disorders that are characterized by dry, thickened, and scaly skin.

_____   _____   _____   _____

True/False

If the statement is true, write **True** on the line. If the statement is false, write **False** on the line.

12.61. _____ An actinic keratosis is a precancerous skin growth that occurs on sun-damaged skin.

12.62. _____ A skin tag is a malignant skin enlargement commonly found on the elderly.

12.63. _____ The arrector pili cause the raised areas of skin known as goose bumps.

12.64. _____ A keratosis is abnormally raised scar.

12.65. _____ Lipedema, which is also known as painful fat syndrome, affects mostly women.

Clinical Conditions

Write the correct answer on the line provided.

12.66. Carmella Espinoza underwent _____ for the treatment of spider veins.

12.67. Jordan Caswell is an albino. This disorder, which is known as _____ , is due to a missing enzyme necessary for the production of melanin.

12.68. Soon after Ying Li hit his thumb with a hammer, a collection of blood formed beneath the nail. This condition is a subungual _____ .

12.69. Trisha fell off her bicycle and scraped off the superficial layers on skin on her knees. This type of injury is known as a/an _____ .

12.70. Molly Malone had a severe fever and then she developed very small, pinpoint hemorrhages under her skin. The doctor described these as being _____ .

12.71. Many of the children in the Happy Hours Day Care Center required treatment for _____ , which is commonly known as an itch mite. The small itchy bumps and blisters of this infestation were caused by tiny mites that burrow into the top layer of human skin to lay their eggs.

12.72. Dr. Liu treated Jeanette Isenberg's skin cancer with _____ _____ . With this technique, individual layers of cancerous tissue are removed and examined under a microscope one at a time until all cancerous tissue has been removed.

12.73. Mrs. Garrison had cosmetic surgery that is commonly known as a lid lift. The medical term for this surgical treatment is a/an _____ .

12.74. Manuel developed a/an _____ . This condition is a closed pocket containing pus that is caused by a bacterial infection.

12.75. Agnes Farrington calls them night sweats; however, the medical term for this condition is

_____   _____ .

Which Is the Correct Medical Term?

Select the correct answer and write it on the line provided.

12.76. The term that refers to an acute infection of the fold of skin at the margin of a nail is

_____ .

onychia   onychocryptosis   paronychia   vitiligo

12.77. When the sebum plug of a _____ is exposed to air, it oxidizes and becomes a blackhead.

chloasma   comedo   macule   pustule

12.78. The condition known as _____ is a common skin disorder characterized by flare-ups in which red papules covered with silvery scales occur on the elbows, knees, scalp, back, or buttocks.

chloasma   miliaria   psoriasis   rosacea

12.79. The medical term referring to a malformation of the nail is _____ . This condition is also called spoon nail.

clubbing   koilonychia   onychomycosis   paronychia

12.80. Commonly known as moles, _____ are small, dark, skin growths that develop from melanocytes in the skin.

keloids   nevi   papillomas   verrucae

Challenge Word Building

These terms are *not* found in this chapter; however, they are made up of the following familiar word parts. If you need help in creating the term, refer to your medical dictionary.

an-	dermat/o	-ia
hypo-	hidr/o	-ectomy
	melan/o	-itis
	myc/o	-malacia
	onych/o	-oma
	py/o	-derma
	rhin/o	-osis
		-pathy
		-plasty

12.81. Abnormal softening of the nails is known as _____ .

12.82. An abnormal condition resulting in the diminished flow of perspiration is known as

_____ .

12.83. The plastic surgery procedure to change the shape or size of the nose is a/an _____ .

12.84. A tumor arising from the nail bed is known as _____ .

12.85. The term meaning any disease marked by abnormal pigmentation of the skin is

_____ .

12.86. The surgical removal of a finger or toenail is a/an _____ .

12.87. The term meaning pertaining to the absence of finger or toenails is _____ .

12.88. The term meaning any disease of the skin is _____ .

12.89. Any disease caused by a fungus is _____ .

12.90. An excess of melanin present in an area of inflammation of the skin is known as

_____ .

Labeling Exercises

Identify the lesions (numbered items) on the accompanying figures.

12.91. _____

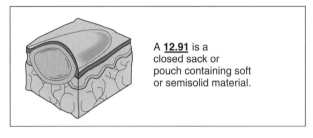

A **12.91** is a closed sack or pouch containing soft or semisolid material.

12.95. _____

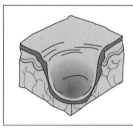

A **12.95** is an open sore or lesion of the skin or mucous membrane resulting in tissue loss.

12.92. _____

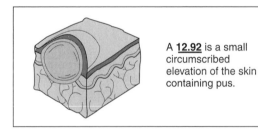

A **12.92** is a small circumscribed elevation of the skin containing pus.

12.96. _____ layer

12.97. _____ layer

12.98. _____ tissue

12.99. _____ gland

12.100. _____ gland

12.93. _____

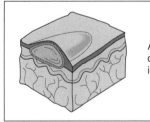

A **12.93** is a small blister containing watery fluid that is less than 0.5 cm in diameter.

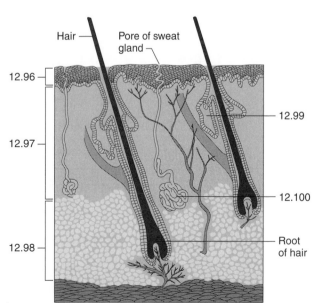

Hair   Pore of sweat gland

12.96 —

12.97 —

12.98 —

12.99

12.100

Root of hair

12.94. _____

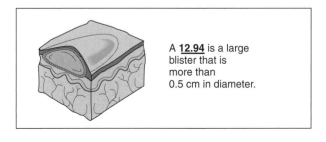

A **12.94** is a large blister that is more than 0.5 cm in diameter.

CHAPTER 13

The Endocrine System

Learning Exercises

Class _____   Name _____

Matching Word Parts 1
Write the correct answer in the middle column.

Definition	Correct Answer	Possible Answers
13.1. adrenal glands	_____	acr/o
13.2. extremities	_____	adren/o
13.3. ovaries or testicles	_____	crin/o
13.4. thirst	_____	-dipsia
13.5. to secrete	_____	gonad/o

Matching Word Parts 2
Write the correct answer in the middle column.

Definition	Correct Answer	Possible Answers
13.6. condition	_____	pituitar/o
13.7. pancreas	_____	pineal/o
13.8. parathyroid	_____	parathyroid/o
13.9. pineal gland	_____	pancreat/o
13.10. pituitary	_____	-ism

Matching Word Parts 3
Write the correct answer in the middle column.

Definition	Correct Answer	Possible Answers
13.11. body	_____	thym/o
13.12. many	_____	thyroid/o
13.13. sugar	_____	somat/o
13.14. thyroid	_____	poly-
13.15. thymus, soul	_____	glyc/o

Definitions

Select the correct answer and write it on the line provided.

13.16. The _____ _____ hormone stimulates ovulation in the female.

    estrogen   follicle-stimulating   lactogenic   luteinizing

13.17. The _____ gland secretes hormones that control the activity of the other endocrine glands.

    adrenal   hypothalamus   pituitary   thymus

13.18. The _____ hormone stimulates the growth and secretions of the adrenal cortex.

    adrenocorticotropic   growth   melanocyte-stimulating   thyroid-stimulating

13.19. The _____ gland has functions in the endocrine and immune systems.

    adrenal   parathyroid   pineal   thymus

13.20. The hormone _____ works with the parathyroid hormone to regulate calcium levels in the blood and tissues.

    aldosterone   calcitonin   glucagon   leptin

13.21. Cortisol is secreted by the _____ _____ .

    adrenal cortex   adrenal medulla   pituitary gland   thyroid gland

13.22. The amount of glucose in the bloodstream is increased by the hormone _____ .

    adrenaline   glucagon   hydrocortisone   insulin

13.23. Norepinephrine is secreted by the _____ _____ .

    adrenal cortex   adrenal medulla   pancreatic islets   pituitary gland

13.24. The hormone _____ stimulates uterine contractions during childbirth.

    estrogen   oxytocin   progesterone   testosterone

13.25. The development of the male secondary sex characteristics is stimulated by the hormone _____ .

    parathyroid   pitocin   progesterone   testosterone

Matching Structures

Write the correct answer in the middle column.

Definition	Correct Answer	Possible Answers
13.26. controls blood sugar levels	_____	thyroid gland
13.27. controls the activity of other endocrine glands	_____	pituitary gland
13.28. influences the sleep-wakefulness cycle	_____	pineal gland
13.29. regulates electrolyte levels	_____	pancreatic islets
13.30. stimulates metabolism	_____	adrenal glands

Which Word?

Select the correct answer and write it on the line provided.

13.31. The hormonal disorder that results from too much growth hormone in adults is known as

_____ .

    acromegaly   gigantism

13.32. The growth hormone is secreted by the _____ _____ of the pituitary gland.

    anterior lobe   posterior lobe

13.33. Diabetes type 2 is an _____ _____ disorder.

    insulin deficiency   insulin resistance

13.34. Insufficient production of ADH causes _____ _____ .

    diabetes insipidus   Graves' disease

13.35. _____ _____ is caused by prolonged exposure to high levels of cortisol.

    Addison's disease   Cushing's syndrome

Spelling Counts

Find the misspelled word in each sentence. Then write that word, spelled correctly, on the line provided.

13.36. Metebolism is the rate at which the body uses energy and the speed at which body functions work.

_____

13.37. Diabetes mellatus is a group of diseases characterized by defects in insulin production, use, or both.

_____

13.38. Myxedemia is also known as adult hypothyroidism. _____

13.39. The hormone progestarone is released during the second half of the menstrual cycle.

_____

13.40. Thymoxin is secreted by the thymus gland.

Abbreviation Identification

In the space provided, write the words that each abbreviation stands for.

13.41. **ACTH** _____

13.42. **ADH** _____

13.43. **DM** _____

13.44. **OGTT** _____

13.45. **FSH** _____

Term Selection

Select the correct answer and write it on the line provided.

13.46. A condition caused by excessive secretion of any gland is known as _____ .

    endocrinopathy   goiter   hypercrinism   hypocrinism

13.47. The condition known as _____ is characterized by abnormally high concentrations of calcium circulating in the blood instead of being stored in the bones.

    hypercalcemia   hyperthyroidism   hypocrinism   polyphagia

13.48. The four _____ glands, each of which is about the size of a grain of rice, are embedded in the posterior surface of the thyroid gland.

    adrenal   pancreatic   parathyroid   pineal

13.49. A/An _____ _____ is a benign tumor of the pituitary gland that causes it to produce too much prolactin.

    insuloma   pheochromocytoma   pituitary adenoma   prolactinoma

13.50. The average blood sugar over the past 3 weeks is measured by the _____

_____ _____ test.

    blood sugar monitoring   fructosamine   glucose tolerance   hemoglobin A1c

Sentence Completion

Write the correct term on the line provided.

13.51. The mineral substances known as _____ are found in the blood and include sodium and potassium.

13.52. The two primary hormones secreted by the thyroid gland are triiodothyronine and

_____ .

13.53. Damage to the retina of the eye caused by diabetes mellitus is known as diabetic

_____ .

13.54. The medical term meaning excessive hunger is _____ .

13.55. Abnormal protrusion of the eye out of the orbit is known as _____ .

Word Surgery

Divide each term into its component word parts. Write these word parts, in sequence, on the lines provided. When necessary use a slash (/) to indicate a combining vowel. (You may not need all of the lines provided.)

13.56. **Hyperpituitarism** is pathology resulting in the excessive secretion by the anterior lobe of the pituitary gland.

_____   _____   _____   _____

13.57. **Hypoglycemia** is an abnormally low concentration of glucose in the blood.

_____   _____   _____   _____

13.58. **Hyperinsulinism** is the condition of excessive secretion of insulin in the bloodstream.

_____   _____   _____   _____

13.59. Gynecomastia is the condition of excessive mammary development in the male.

_____ _____ _____ _____

13.60. Hypocalcemia is characterized by abnormally low levels of calcium in the blood.

_____ _____ _____ _____

True/False

If the statement is true, write **True** on the line. If the statement is false, write **False** on the line.

13.61. _____ The beta cells of the pancreatic islets secrete glucagon in response to low blood sugar levels.

13.62. _____ A pheochromocytoma is a benign tumor of the adrenal medulla that causes the gland to produce excess epinephrine.

13.63. _____ Human chorionic gonadotropin (HCG) is secreted by the adrenal cortex.

13.64. _____ An insulinoma is a malignant tumor of the pancreas that causes hypoglycemia by secreting insulin.

13.65. _____ Polyuria is excessive urination.

Clinical Conditions

Write the correct answer on the line provided.

13.66. During his studies, Rodney Milne learned that the _____ hormone maintains the water balance within the body by promoting the reabsorption of water through the kidneys.

13.67. Eduardo Chavez complained of being thirsty all the time. His doctor noted this excessive thirst on his chart as _____ .

13.68. Mrs. Wei's symptoms included chronic, worsening fatigue and muscle weakness, loss of appetite, and weight loss because her adrenal glands do not produce enough cortisol. Her doctor diagnosed this condition as _____ _____ .

13.69. Linda Thomas was diagnosed as having a/an _____ . This is a benign tumor of the pancreas that causes hypoglycemia by secreting insulin.

13.70. Patrick Edward has the autoimmune disorder known as _____

_____ . In this the body's own antibodies attack and destroy the cells of the thyroid gland.

13.71. When "the champ" was training for the Olympics, he was tempted to use _____ steroids to increase his strength and muscle mass.

13.72. Holly Yates was surprised to learn that _____ , which is a hormone secreted by fat cells, travels to the brain and controls the balance of food intake and energy expenditure.

13.73. As a result of a congenital lack of thyroid secretion, the Vaugh-Eames child suffers from _____ , which is a condition of arrested physical and mental development.

13.74. Ray Grovenor is excessively tall and large. This condition, which was caused by excessive functioning of the pituitary gland before puberty, is known as _____ .

13.75. Rosita DeAngelis required the surgical removal of her pancreas. The medical term for this procedure is a/an _____ .

Which Is the Correct Medical Term?

Select the correct answer and write it on the line provided.

13.76. Although they are produced by specialized cells in the brain, _____ are able to travel through the bloodstream and affect cells throughout distant parts of the body.

hormones	neurohormones	neurotransmitters	steroids

13.77. A/An _____ _____ is a slow-growing, benign tumor of the pituitary gland that is a functioning tumor (secreting hormones) or a nonfunctioning tumor (not secreting hormones).

hyperpituitarism	hypopituitarism	pituitary adenoma	prolactinoma

13.78. _____ disease, which is an autoimmune disorder caused by hyperthyroidism, is characterized by goiter and/or exophthalmos.

Addison's	Cushing's	Graves'	Hashimoto's

13.79. The diabetic emergency caused by very high blood sugar is a/an _____ _____ . This condition must be treated by the prompt administration of insulin.

diabetic coma	hypoglycemia	insulin shock	insuloma

13.80. The hormone _____ , which is secreted by the pineal gland, influences the sleep-wakefulness cycles.

glucagons	melatonin	parathyroid	thymosin

Challenge Word Building

These terms are *not* found in this chapter; however, they are made up of the following familiar word parts. If you need help in creating the term, refer to your medical dictionary.

endo-	adren/o	-emia
	crin/o	-itis
	insulin/o	-megaly
	pancreat/o	-ology
	pineal/o	-oma
	thym/o	-otomy
	thyroid/o	-pathy

13.81. The term meaning any disease of the adrenal glands is _____ .

13.82. The study of endocrine glands and their secretions is known as _____ .

13.83. Abnormal enlargement of the adrenal glands is known as _____ .

13.84. The term meaning any disease of the thymus gland is _____ .

13.85. Inflammation of the thyroid gland is known as _____ .

13.86. A surgical incision into the pancreas is a/an _____ .

13.87. A surgical incision into the thyroid gland is a/an _____ .

13.88. The term meaning any disease of the pineal gland is _____ .

13.89. Abnormally high levels of insulin in the blood are known as _____ .

13.90. Inflammation of the adrenal glands is known as _____ .

Labeling Exercises

Identify the numbered items on the accompanying figure.

13.91. _____ gland

13.92. _____ glands

13.93. _____ gland

13.94. _____ of the female

13.95. _____

13.96. _____ gland

13.97. _____ gland

13.98. _____ glands

13.99. _____ islets

13.100. _____ of the male

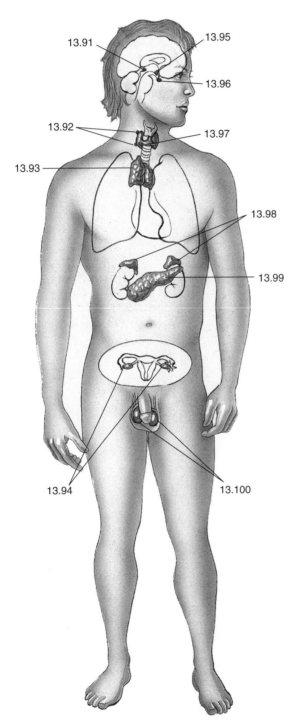

CHAPTER 14

The Reproductive Systems

Learning Exercises

Class _____   Name _____

Matching Word Parts 1
Write the correct answer in the middle column.

Definition	Correct Answer	Possible Answers
14.1. cervix	_____	men/o
14.2. female	_____	gynec/o
14.3. menstruation	_____	-gravida
14.4. pregnant	_____	colp/o
14.5. vagina	_____	cervic/o

Matching Word Parts 2
Write the correct answer in the middle column.

Definition	Correct Answer	Possible Answers
14.6. egg	_____	vagin/o
14.7. ovary	_____	test/i, test/o
14.8. testicle	_____	ov/o
14.9. uterus	_____	ovari/o
14.10. vagina	_____	hyster/o

Matching Word Parts 3
Write the correct answer in the middle column.

Definition	Correct Answer	Possible Answers
14.11. breast	_____	salping/o
14.12. none	_____	-pexy
14.13. surgical fixation	_____	-para
14.14. to bring forth	_____	nulli-
14.15. tube	_____	mast/o

Definitions

Select the correct answer and write it on the line provided.

14.16. The term that describes the inner layer of the uterus is _____ .

    corpus   endometrium   myometrium   perimetrium

14.17. The term describing the single cells formed immediately after conception is known as a/an

    _____ .

    embryo   fetus   gamete   zygote

14.18. The mucus that lubricates the vagina is produced by the _____

    _____ .

    Bartholin's glands   bulbourethral glands   Cowper's glands   hymen glands

14.19. The finger-like structures of the fallopian tube that catch the ovum are the

    _____ .

    fimbriae   fundus   infundibulum   oviducts

14.20. The term _____ is used to designate the transition phase between regular menstrual periods and no periods at all.

    menarche   menopause   perimenopause   puberty

14.21. The medical term for the condition also known as vaginal thrush or a yeast infection is

    _____ _____ .

    colporrhea   leukorrhea   pruritus vulvae   vaginal candidiasis

14.22. Sperm are formed within the _____ _____ of each testicle.

    ejaculatory ducts   epididymis   seminiferous tubules   urethra

14.23. During puberty, the term _____ describes the beginning of the menstrual function.

    menarche   menopause   menses   menstruation

14.24. In the female, the region between the vaginal orifice and the anus is known as the

    _____ _____ .

    clitoris   mons pubis   perineum   vulva

14.25. The release of a mature egg by the ovary is known as _____ .

    coitus   fertilization   menstruation   ovulation

Matching Structures

Write the correct answer in the middle column.

Definition	Correct Answer	Possible Answers
14.26. carry milk from the mammary glands	_____	vulva
14.27. encloses the testicles	_____	scrotum
14.28. external female genitalia	_____	lactiferous ducts
14.29. protects the tip of the penis	_____	foreskin
14.30. sensitive tissue near the vaginal opening	_____	clitoris

Which Word?

Select the correct answer and write it on the line provided.

14.31. The term used to describe a woman during her first pregnancy is a _____ .

    primigravida   primipara

14.32. The fluid secreted by the breasts during the first days after giving birth is _____ .

    colostrum   meconium

14.33. The term _____ describes an inflammation of the cervix that is usually caused by an infection.

    cervicitis   vulvitis

14.34. From implantation through the 8th week of pregnancy, the developing child is known as a/an

_____ .

    embryo   fetus

14.35. A _____ is a woman who has never borne a viable child.

    nulligravida   nullipara

Spelling Counts

Find the misspelled word in each sentence. Then write that word, spelled correctly, on the line provided.

14.36. The prostrate gland secretes a thick fluid that aids the motility of the sperm. _____

14.37. The normal periodic discharge from the uterus is known as menstration. _____

14.38. The third stage of labor and delivery is the expulsion of the plasenta is delivered as the afterbirth.

_____

14.39. The term hemaspermia is the presence of blood in the seminal fluid. _____

14.40. The surgical removal of the foreskin of the penis is known as cercumsion. _____

Abbreviation Identification

In the space provided, write the words that each abbreviation stands for.

14.41. **AMA** _____

14.42. **PID** _____

14.43. **PMDD** _____

14.44. **Trich** _____

14.45. **VD** _____

Term Selection

Select the correct answer and write it on the line provided.

14.46. An accumulation of pus in the fallopian tube is known as _____

_____ .

    oophoritis   pelvic inflammatory disease   pyosalpinx   salpingitis

14.47. A _____ is a knot of varicose veins in one side of the scrotum.

hydrocele   phimosis   priapism   varicocele

14.48. The direct visual examination of the tissues of the cervix and vagina using a binocular magnifier is

known as _____ _____ .

colposcopy   endovaginal ultrasound   hysteroscopy   laparoscopy

14.49. The term used to describe infrequent or very light menstruation in a woman with previously normal

periods is _____ .

amenorrhea   hypomenorrhea   oligomenorrhea   polymenorrhea

14.50. The examination of cells retrieved from the edge of the placenta between the eighth and tenth weeks of

pregnancy is known as _____ _____ _____ .

amniocentesis   chorionic villus sampling   fetal monitoring   pelvimetry

Sentence Completion

Write the correct term on the line provided.

14.51. The dark area surrounding the nipple is known as the _____ .

14.52. A fluid-filled sac in the scrotum along the spermatic cord leading from the testicles is known as a/an

_____ .

14.53. The serious complication of pregnancy that is characterized by convulsions and sometimes coma is

known as _____ . The treatment for this condition is delivery of the fetus.

14.54. Surgical suturing of a tear in the vagina is known as _____ .

14.55. The _____ _____ is the tube that carries blood, oxygen, and

nutrients from the placenta to the developing child.

Word Surgery

Divide each term into its component word parts. Write these word parts, in sequence, on the lines provided.
When necessary use a slash (/) to indicate a combining vowel. (You may not need all of the lines provided.)

14.56. **Endocervicitis** is an inflammation of the mucous membrane lining of the cervix.

_____   _____   _____   _____

14.57. **Menometrorrhagia** is excessive uterine bleeding at both the usual time of menstrual periods and at
other irregular intervals.

_____   _____   _____   _____

14.58. **Hysterosalpingography** is a specialized radiographic examination of the uterus and fallopian tubes.

_____   _____   _____   _____

14.59. **Anorchism** is the absence of one or both testicles. This condition can be congenital or acquired.

_____   _____   _____   _____

14.60. **Azoospermia** is the absence of sperm in the semen.

_____   _____   _____   _____

True/False

If the statement is true, write **True** on the line. If the statement is false, write **False** on the line.

14.61. _____ Peyronie's disease causes a sexual dysfunction in which the penis is bent or curved during erection.

14.62. _____ Braxton Hicks contractions are the first true labor pains.

14.63. _____ An Apgar score is an evaluation of a newborn infant's physical status at 1 and 5 minutes after birth.

14.64. _____ Breast augmentation is mammoplasty that is performed to reduce breast size.

14.65. _____ An ectopic pregnancy is a potentially dangerous condition in which a fertilized egg is implanted and begins to develop outside of the uterus.

Clinical Conditions

Write the correct answer on the line provided.

14.66. Baby Ortega was born with cryptorchidism. When this testicle had not descended by the time he was 9 months old, a/an _____ was performed to move an undescended testicle into its normal position in the scrotum.

14.67. When she went into labor with her first child, Mrs. Hoshi's baby was in a breech presentation. Because of risks associated with this, her obstetrician delivered the baby surgically by performing a/an _____ _____ .

14.68. Dawn Grossman was diagnosed as having uterine fibroids that required surgical removal. Her gynecologist scheduled Dawn for a/an _____ .

14.69. Rita Chen, who is 25 years old and knows that she is not pregnant, is concerned because she has not had a menstrual period for 3 months. Her doctor described this condition as _____ .

14.70. Enrico's physician removed a portion of each vas deferens. The medical term for this sterilization procedure is a/an _____ .

14.71. Tiffany developed a thin, frothy, yellow-green, foul-smelling vaginal discharge. She was diagnosed as having the venereal disease known as _____ , which is caused by the protozoan parasite *Trichomonas vaginalis*.

14.72. Mr. Wolford, who is age 65, has been reading a lot about male menopause. His physician told him that the medical term for this condition is _____ .

14.73. Just before the delivery of her baby, Barbara Klein's obstetrician performed a/an _____ to prevent tearing of the tissues as the child moved through the birth canal.

14.74. Jane Marsall's pregnancy was complicated by the abnormal implantation of the placenta in the lower portion of the uterus. The medical term for this condition is _____ .

14.75. Immediately after birth, the Reicher baby was described as being a newborn or a/an _____ .

Which Is the Correct Medical Term?

Select the correct answer and write it on the line provided.

14.76. The post-partum vaginal discharge during the first several week after childbirth is known as

_____ .

colostrum   involution   lochia   meconium

14.77. Abdominal pain caused by uterine cramps during a menstrual period is known as

_____ .

dysmenorrhea   hypermenorrhea   menometrorrhagia   polymenorrhea

14.78. The term that describes an inflammation of the glans penis is _____ .

anorchism   balanitis   epididymitis   testitis

14.79. An inflammation of the lining of the vagina is known as _____ . The most common causes of this condition are bacterial vaginosis, trichomoniasis, and vaginal candidiasis.

cervical dysplasia   cervicitis   colporrhexis   vaginitis

14.80. The term that describes a profuse white mucus discharge from the uterus and vagina is

_____ . This type of discharge can be due to an infection, malignancy, or hormonal changes.

endocervicitis   leukorrhea   pruritus vulvae   vaginitis

Challenge Word Building

These terms are *not* found in this chapter; however, they are made up of the following familiar word parts. If you need help in creating the term, refer to your medical dictionary.

endo-	hyster/o	-cele
	mast/o	-dynia
	metr/i	-itis
	oophor/o	-pexy
	orchid/o	-plasty
	vagin/o	-rrhaphy
	vulv/o	-rrhexis

14.81. The term meaning a hernia protruding into the vagina is _____ .

14.82. The term meaning the surgical repair of one or both testicles is _____ .

14.83. The term meaning an inflammation of the endometrium is _____ .

14.84. The term meaning the surgical repair of an ovary is a/an _____ .

14.85. The term meaning pain in the vagina is _____ .

11.86. The term meaning surgical suturing of the uterus is _____ .

14.87. The term meaning a hernia of the uterus, particularly during pregnancy, is a/an

_____ .

14.88. The term meaning the surgical fixation of a displaced ovary is _____ .

14.89. The term meaning the rupture of the uterus, particularly during pregnancy, is

_____ .

14.90. The term meaning an inflammation of the vulva and the vagina is _____ .

Labeling Exercises
Identify the numbered items on these accompanying figures.

14.91. _____ bladder

14.92. _____ gland

14.93. _____

14.94. _____

14.95. _____

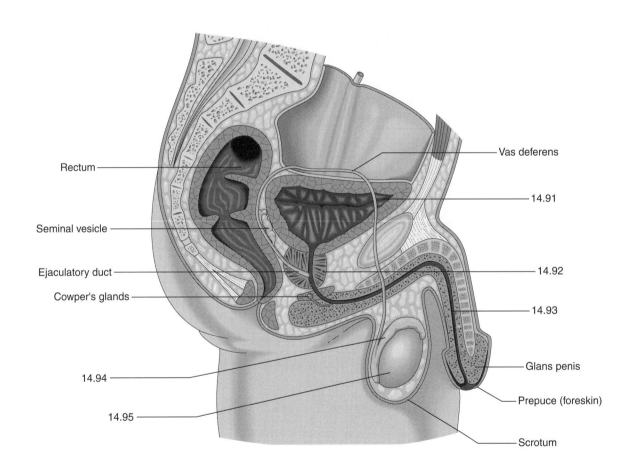

14.96. _____ or uterine tube

14.97. body of the _____

14.98. _____ bladder

14.99. _____

14.100. _____

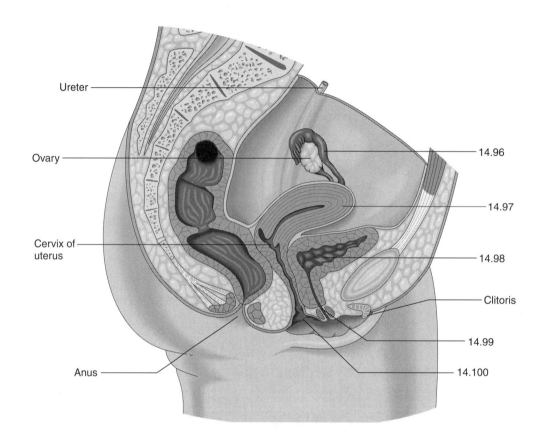

Diagnostic Procedures and Pharmacology

Learning Exercises

Class _____   Name _____

Matching Word Parts 1
Write the correct answer in the middle column.

Definition	Correct Answer	Possible Answers
15.1. abdomen	_____	lapar/o
15.2. albumin, protein	_____	glycos/o
15.3. calcium	_____	creatin/o
15.4. creatinine	_____	calc/i
15.5. sugar	_____	albumin/o

Matching Word Parts 2
Write the correct answer in the middle column.

Definition	Correct Answer	Possible Answers
15.6. surgical puncture for the removal of fluid	_____	son/o
15.7. blood	_____	-otomy
15.8. surgical incision	_____	hemat/o
15.9. process of producing a picture or record	_____	-graphy
15.10. sound	_____	-centesis

Matching Word Parts 3

Write the correct answer in the middle column.

Definition	Correct Answer	Possible Answers
15.11. direct visual examination	_____	-uria
15.12. radiation	_____	-scopy
15.13. urine	_____	-scope
15.14. vein	_____	radi/o
15.15. visual examination instrument	_____	phleb/o

Definitions

Select the correct answer and write it on the line provided.

15.16. In radiography, a/an _____ projection has the patient positioned at right angles to the film.

   anteroposterior   lateral   oblique   posteroanterior

15.17. A/An _____ is used to enlarge the opening of any body canal or cavity to facilitate inspection of its interior.

   endoscope   otoscope   speculum   sphygmomanometer

15.18. The imaging technique that produces multiple cross-sectional images using x-radiation is

   _____ _____ _____ .

   computed tomography   fluoroscopy   magnetic resonance imaging   radiography

15.19. A/An _____ _____ test a screening test to evaluate platelet function and to monitor changes in the blood associated with chemotherapy and radiation therapy.

   basic metabolic panel   erythrocyte sedimentation hematocrit   platelet count

15.20. The diagnostic technique _____ _____ creates images of deep body structures by recording the echoes of pulses of sound waves that are above the range of human hearing.

   cineradiography   extraoral radiography   fluoroscopy   ultrasonography

15.21. The presence of calcium in the urine is known as _____ .

   albuminuria   calciuria   creatinuria   glycosuria

15.22. A/An _____ _____ test is used to monitor anticoagulant therapy. It is performed to identify high levels of inflammation within the body.

   blood urea nitrogen   C-reactive protein   erythrocyte sedimentation   serum bilirubin

15.23. In the _____ _____ position, the patient is lying on the back with the knees bent.

   dorsal recumbent   horizontal recumbent   knee-chest   supine

15.24. A _____ is an abnormal sound heard during of auscultation of an artery.

   bruit   rale   rhonchus   stridor

15.25. The substance, which has a sweet, fruity odor, that is found in small quantities in normal urine and in larger amount in diabetic urine is _____ .

   acetone   creatinine   ketone   urea

Matching Techniques
Write the correct answer in the middle column.

Definition	Correct Answer	Possible Answers
15.26. produces cross-sectional views	_____	x-rays
15.27. produces views in only one direction	_____	MRI
15.28. the removal of fluid for diagnostic purposes	_____	fluoroscopy
15.29. uses a glowing screen	_____	centesis
15.30. uses powerful magnets	_____	CT

Which Word?
Select the correct answer and write it on the line provided.

15.31. A/An _____ reaction is an unexpected reaction to a drug that is peculiar to the individual.

    idiosyncratic   palliative

15.32. _____ _____ _____

_____ tomography combines tomography with radionuclide tracers to produce enhanced images of selected body organs or areas.

    Positron emission   Single photon emission computed

15.33. A substance that does not allow x-rays to pass through is described as being

_____ .

    radiolucent   radiopaque

15.34. A bitewing dental film is an example of _____ radiography.

    extraoral   intraoral

15.35. A _____ _____ drug is sold under the name given the drug by the manufacturer. These drug names are always spelled with a capital letter.

    brand name   generic

Spelling Counts
Find the misspelled word in each sentence. Then write that word, spelled correctly, on the line provided.

15.36. Listening through a stethoscope for sounds within the body to determine the condition of the lungs, pleura, heart, and abdomen is known as asultation. _____

15.37. A sphygnomanometer is used to measure blood pressure. _____

15.38. Fluroscopy is the visualization of body parts in motion by projecting x-ray images on a luminous fluorescent screen. _____

15.39. A conterindication is a factor in the patient's condition that makes the use of a medication or specific treatment dangerous or ill advised. _____

15.40. An opthalmoscope is used to examine the interior of the eye. _____

Abbreviation Identification

In the space provided, write the words that each abbreviation stands for.

15.41. **ESR** _____

15.42. **NPO** _____

15.43. **p.r.n.** _____

15.44. **TPR** _____

15.45. **WBC** _____

Term Selection

Select the correct answer and write it on the line provided.

15.46. Drawing fluid from the sac surrounding the heart is known as _____ .

    abdominocentesis   cardiocentesis   pericardiocentesis   tympanocentesis

15.47. The abnormal presence of blood in the urine is known as _____ .

    albuminuria   creatinuria   hematuria   ketonuria

15.48. A/An _____ projection has the patient positioned with the back parallel to the film.

    anteroposterior   lateral   oblique   posteroanterior

15.49. A/An _____ relieves inflammation and pain without affecting consciousness.

    acetaminophen   analgesic   anti-inflammatory   palliative

15.50. The term _____ means the administration of a medication by injection.

    hypodermic   parenteral   transcutaneous   transdermal

Sentence Completion

Write the correct term on the line provided.

15.51. The term radiographic _____ describes the path that the x-ray beam follows through the body from entrance to exit.

15.52. The term _____ describes an abnormal, high-pitched harsh or crowing sound that is heard during inspiration.

15.53. A/An _____ is an individual trained and skilled in drawing blood to be tested.

15.54. A/An _____ is an instrument used to visually examine the external ear and the eardrum.

15.55. A/An _____ is compulsive, uncontrollable dependence on a substance, habit, or practice to the degree that stopping causes severe emotional, mental, or physiologic reactions.

Word Surgery

Divide each term into its component word parts. Write these word parts, in sequence, on the lines provided. When necessary use a slash (/) to indicate a combining vowel. (You may not need all of the lines provided.)

15.56. **Tympanocentesis** is the surgical puncture of the tympanic membrane with a needle to remove fluid from the middle ear.

_____   _____   _____   _____

15.57. **Cineradiography** is the recording of images as they appear in motion on a fluorescent screen.

_____   _____   _____   _____

15.58. **Echocardiography** is an ultrasonic diagnostic procedure used to evaluate the structures and motion of the heart.

_____ _____ _____ _____

15.59. **Bacteriuria** is the presence of bacteria in the urine.

_____ _____ _____ _____

15.60. **Pharmacology** is the study of the nature, uses, and effects of drugs for medical purposes.

_____ _____ _____ _____

True/False

If the statement is true, write **True** on the line. If the statement is false, write **False** on the line.

15.61. _____ An oblique projection has the patient's body positioned parallel to the film.

15.62. _____ Casts are fibrous or protein materials, such as pus and fats, that are thrown off into the urine in kidney disease.

15.63. _____ A placebo has the potential to cure a disease.

15.64. _____ An MRI creates images by combining high-frequency ultrasonic waves and strong magnets.

15.65. _____ Compliance means that the patient has accurately followed instructions.

Clinical Conditions

Write the correct answer on the line provided.

15.66. The urinalysis for Sophia showed the presence of pus. The medical term for this condition is

_____ .

15.67. Dr. Jamison suspected her patient had an infection. An elevated count in the patient's

_____ _____ cell count test would confirm her diagnosis.

15.68. Kelly Harrison was extremely cold after being stranded in a snow storm. When rescued, the

paramedics said she was suffering from _____ .

15.69. During his examination of the patient, Dr. Wong used _____ to feel the texture, size, consistency, and location of certain body parts.

15.70. Dr. McDowell ordered a blood transfusion. Before the transfusion _____ , tests were required to determine the compatibility of donor's and recipient's blood.

15.71. In preparation for his upper GI series, Dwight Oshone swallowed a liquid containing the contrast

medium _____ .

15.72. Maria Martinez required _____ echocardiography (TEE) to evaluate the structures of her heart.

15.73. In preparation for his back examination, Scott Cunningham was placed in a _____ position. Scott was lying on his belly with his face down and his arms were placed under his head for comfort.

15.74. The urinalysis for Kathleen McCaffee showed _____ . This is the presence of glucose in the urine.

15.75. Dr. Roberts used _____ during the examination. This technique involves tapping the surface of the body with a finger or instrument.

Which Is the Correct Medical Term?

Select the correct answer and write it on the line provided.

15.76. A/An _____ drug reaction is an undesirable reaction that accompanies the principal response for which the drug was taken.

   adverse   idiosyncratic   potentiation   synergism

15.77. The urinalysis indicated _____ . This is an increased concentration of creatinine in the urine.

   creatinuria   glycosuria   ketonuria   proteinuria

15.78. A/An _____ dental radiograph shows the entire tooth and some of the surrounding tissue.

   bite-wing   extraoral   periapical   survey

15.79. During a _____ examination, some patients feel uncomfortable because of the noise generated by the machine and the feeling of being closed in.

   CT   MRI   PET   x-ray

15.80. The examination position that has the patient in a supine position with the feet and legs supported in stirrups is the _____ _____ position.

   dorsal recumbent   lithotomy   prone   Sims'

Challenge Word Building

These terms are *not* found in this chapter; however, they are made up of the following familiar word parts. If you need help in creating the term, refer to your medical dictionary.

   hyper-   albumin/o   -centesis
   hypo-   calc/i   -emia
                       cyst/o   -scope
                       glycos/o   -uria
                       protein/o
                       pleur/o
                       py/o

15.81. The term meaning the presence of abnormally low concentrations of protein in the blood is

   _____ .

15.82. The term meaning abnormally high levels of albumin in the blood is _____ .

15.83. The term meaning unusually large amounts of sugar in the urine is _____ .

15.84. The instrument used to visually examine the interior of the urinary bladder is a/an

   _____ .

15.85. The term meaning the presence of pus in excreted urine is _____ .

15.86. The term meaning a surgical puncture of the chest wall with a needle to obtain fluid from the pleural cavity is _____ . This procedure is also known as thoracentesis.

15.87. The term meaning an abnormally low level of calcium in the circulating blood is

   _____ .

15.88. The term meaning abnormally large amounts of calcium in the urine is _____ .

15.89. The term meaning the presence of pus-forming organisms in the blood is _____ .

15.90. The term meaning the presence of excess protein in the urine is _____ .

Labeling Exercises

Identify the numbered items on the accompanying figures.

15.91.   This is the _____ position.

15.92.   This is the _____ recumbent position.

15.93.   This is the _____ position.

15.94.   This is the _____ recumbent position.

15.95.   This is the _____ position.

15.96.   This is the _____ position.

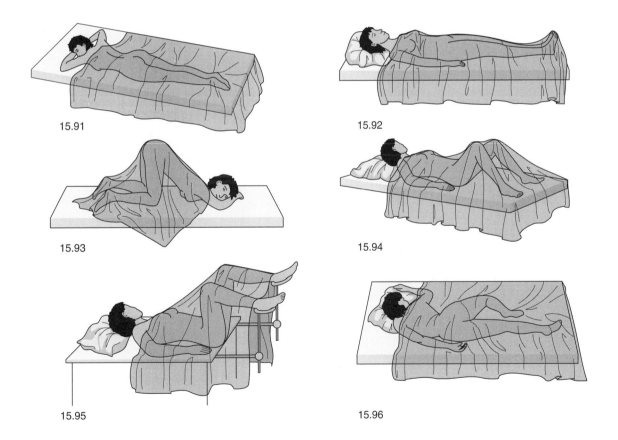

15.91

15.92

15.93

15.94

15.95

15.96

15.97.   This is a/an _____ injection.

15.98.   This is a/an _____ injection.

15.99.   This is a/an _____ injection.

15.100. This is a/an _____ injection.

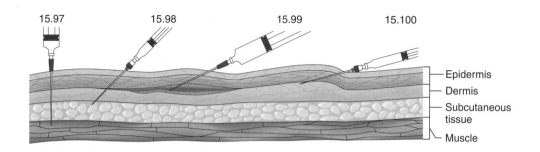

Comprehensive Medical Terminology Review

Overview of Comprehensive Medical Terminology Review

Study Tips

Hints to help you review more effectively.

Answer Sheets

Write the *letter* of the correct answer for the questions in the review tests. Although only one set of answer sheets are included, you can take these tests as often as you want.

Review Session

A 100-multiple-choice question Review Session to help you determine where you need more study emphasis. However, be aware that none of these questions is from the actual final test.

Simulated Medical Terminology Final Test

A 100-multiple-choice question "mock" final test to help you evaluate your progress. The "Simulated Medical Terminology Final Test." However, be aware that none of these questions is from the actual final test.

STUDY TIPS

Use Your Vocabulary Lists

- Photocopy the vocabulary list for each chapter in your textbook and add any terms suggested by your instructor. This creates a study aid that is easy to carry with you for additional review whenever you have a free minute.

- Review the terms on each list. When you have mastered a term, put a check in the box next to it. If you cannot spell and define a term, highlight it for further study.

- Look up the meanings of the highlighted terms in the textbook and work on mastering them.

- When using a list isn't convenient, consider listening to the **Audio CDs** that accompany this text.

- Caution: Do not limit your studying to these lists. Although they contain important terms, there are many additional important words in each chapter that you need to know.

Use Your Flash Cards

- Use the flash cards from the back of this book.

- As you go through them, remove from the stack all those word parts you can define.

- Keep working until you have mastered all of these word parts.

Make Your Own Study List

- By now you should have greatly reduced the number of terms still to be mastered. Make a list of these terms and word parts, and concentrate on them.

Review Your Learning Exercises

- As your corrected Learning Exercises are returned, save them. At review time, go through these sheets and make a note of where you have made mistakes. Ask yourself, *"Do I know the correct answer now?"* If it is not correct, add the term or word part to your study list.

Help Someone Else

- One of the greatest ways to really learn something is to teach it! If a classmate is having trouble, tutoring that person will help both of you learn the material.

Use the Practice Sessions

- The next two pages are answer sheets to be used with the "Review Session" and "Simulated Medical Terminology Final Test" that follow.

Review Session Answer Sheet

Write a **letter** of the correct answer on the line next to the question number.

Class _____   **Name** _____

RS.1. _____	RS.26. _____	RS.51. _____	RS.76. _____
RS.2. _____	RS.27. _____	RS.52. _____	RS.77. _____
RS.3. _____	RS.28. _____	RS.53. _____	RS.78. _____
RS.4. _____	RS.29. _____	RS.54. _____	RS.79. _____
RS.5. _____	RS.30. _____	RS.55. _____	RS.80. _____
RS.6. _____	RS.31. _____	RS.56. _____	RS.81. _____
RS.7. _____	RS.32. _____	RS.57. _____	RS.82. _____
RS.8. _____	RS.33. _____	RS.58. _____	RS.83. _____
RS.9. _____	RS.34. _____	RS.59. _____	RS.84. _____
RS.10. _____	RS.35. _____	RS.60. _____	RS.85. _____
RS.11. _____	RS.36. _____	RS.61. _____	RS.86. _____
RS.12. _____	RS.37. _____	RS.62. _____	RS.87. _____
RS.13. _____	RS.38. _____	RS.63. _____	RS.88. _____
RS.14. _____	RS.39. _____	RS.64. _____	RS.89. _____
RS.15. _____	RS.40. _____	RS.65. _____	RS.90. _____
RS.16. _____	RS.41. _____	RS.66. _____	RS.91. _____
RS.17. _____	RS.42. _____	RS.67. _____	RS.92. _____
RS.18. _____	RS.43. _____	RS.68. _____	RS.93. _____
RS.19. _____	RS.44. _____	RS.69. _____	RS.94. _____
RS.20. _____	RS.45. _____	RS.70. _____	RS.95. _____
RS.21. _____	RS.46. _____	RS.71. _____	RS.96. _____
RS.22. _____	RS.47. _____	RS.72. _____	RS.97. _____
RS.23. _____	RS.48. _____	RS.73. _____	RS.98. _____
RS.24. _____	RS.49. _____	RS.74. _____	RS.99. _____
RS.25. _____	RS.50. _____	RS.75. _____	RS.100. _____

Simulated Medical Terminology Final

Test Answer Sheet

Write a **letter** of the correct answer on the line next to the question number.

Class _____   Name _____

FT.1. _____   FT.26. _____   FT.51. _____   FT.76. _____

FT.2. _____   FT.27. _____   FT.52. _____   FT.77. _____

FT.3. _____   FT.28. _____   FT.53. _____   FT.78. _____

FT.4. _____   FT.29. _____   FT.54. _____   FT.79. _____

FT.5. _____   FT.30. _____   FT.55. _____   FT.80. _____

FT.6. _____   FT.31. _____   FT.56. _____   FT.81. _____

FT.7. _____   FT.32. _____   FT.57. _____   FT.82. _____

FT.8. _____   FT.33. _____   FT.58. _____   FT.83. _____

FT.9. _____   FT.34. _____   FT.59. _____   FT.84. _____

FT.10. _____   FT.35. _____   FT.60. _____   FT.85. _____

FT.11. _____   FT.36. _____   FT.61. _____   FT.86. _____

FT.12. _____   FT.37. _____   FT.62. _____   FT.87. _____

FT.13. _____   FT.38. _____   FT.63. _____   FT.88. _____

FT.14. _____   FT.39. _____   FT.64. _____   FT.89. _____

FT.15. _____   FT.40. _____   FT.65. _____   FT.90. _____

FT.16. _____   FT.41. _____   FT.66. _____   FT.91. _____

FT.17. _____   FT.42. _____   FT.67. _____   FT.92. _____

FT.18. _____   FT.43. _____   FT.68. _____   FT.93. _____

FT.19. _____   FT.44. _____   FT.69. _____   FT.94. _____

FT.20. _____   FT.45. _____   FT.70. _____   FT.95. _____

FT.21. _____   FT.46. _____   FT.71. _____   FT.96. _____

FT.22. _____   FT.47. _____   FT.72. _____   FT.97. _____

FT.23. _____   FT.48. _____   FT.73. _____   FT.98. _____

FT.24. _____   FT.49. _____   FT.74. _____   FT.99. _____

FT.25. _____   FT.50. _____   FT.75. _____   FT.100. _____

Review Session

RS.1. An abnormally rapid rate of respiration of more than 20 breaths per minute is known as _____ .

a. bradypnea

b. eupnea

c. hyperventilation

d. tachypnea

RS.2. An abnormally slow heart rate of less than 60 beats per minute is known as _____ .

a. atrial fibrillation

b. bradycardia

c. palpitation

d. tachycardia

RS.3. The suffix _____ means surgical fixation.

a. -desis

b. -lysis

c. -pexy

d. -ptosis

RS.4. The presence of glucose in the urine is known as _____ .

a. albuminuria

b. calciuria

c. glycosuria

d. hematuria

RS.5. A collection of pus within a body cavity is known as a/an _____ .

a. cyst

b. empyema

c. hernia

d. tumor

RS.6. An _____ is the surgical removal of a joint.

a. angiectomy

b. arteriectomy

c. atherectomy

d. arthrectomy

RS.7. The abnormal development or growth of cells is known as _____ .

a. anaplasia

b. dysplasia

c. hyperplasia

d. hypertrophy

RS.8. Which form of anemia is a genetic disorder.

a. aplastic

b. hemolytic

c. megaloblastic

d. sickle cell

RS.9. The medical term for the condition commonly known as brown lung disease is _____ .

a. anthracosis

b. byssinosis

c. pneumoconiosis

d. silicosis

RS.10. _____ is an inflammation of the myelin sheath of peripheral nerves, characterized by rapidly worsening muscle weakness that can lead to temporary paralysis.

a. Bell's palsy

b. Guillain-Barré syndrome

c. Lou Gehrig's disease

d. Raynaud's phenomenon

RS.11. The term _____ describes weakness or wearing away of body tissues and structures caused by pathology or by disuse of the muscle over a long period of time.

a. adhesion

b. ankylosis

c. atrophy

d. contracture

RS.12. The suffix _____ means blood or blood condition.

a. -emia

b. -oma

c. -pnea

d. -uria

RS.13. The procedure in which an anastomosis is created between the upper portion of the stomach and the duodenum is a/an _____ .

    a. esophagogastrectomy

    b. esophagoplasty

    c. gastroduodenostomy

    d. gastrostomy

RS.14. The term _____ , which is also known as wheezing, is the sound heard during breathing out as air passes out through a partially obstructed airway.

    a. bruit

    b. rale

    c. rhonchus

    d. stridor

RS.15. The term _____ means abnormal enlargement of the liver.

    a. hepatitis

    b. hepatomalacia

    c. hepatomegaly

    d. hepatorrhexis

RS.16. The term describing the prolapse of a kidney is _____ .

    a. nephrectasis

    b. nephroptosis

    c. nephropyosis

    d. nephropexy

RS.17. Which of these conditions is commonly known as a bruise?

    a. ecchymosis

    b. epistaxis

    c. hematoma

    d. lesion

RS.18. The acute respiratory syndrome known as _____ , is characterized in children and infants by obstruction of the larynx, hoarseness, and a barking cough.

    a. asthma

    b. croup

    c. diphtheria

    d. pneumonia

RS.19. _____ is a condition in which the immune system mistakenly attacks and progressively destroys the thyroid gland.

    a. Conn's disease

    b. Hashimoto's thyroiditis

    c. Lou Gehrig's disease

    d. Grave's disease

RS.20. Which sexually transmitted disease can be detected through the VDRL blood test before the lesions appear?

    a. chlamydia

    b. gonorrhea

    c. syphilis

    d. trichomoniasis

RS.21. A blood clot attached to the interior wall of a vein or artery is known as a/an _____ .

    a. embolism

    b. embolus

    c. thrombosis

    d. thrombus

RS.22. The term _____ describes the removal of a body part or the destruction of its function by surgery, hormones, drugs, heat, chemical destruction, electrocautery, or other methods.

    a. ablation

    b. abrasion

    c. cryosurgery

    d. exfoliative cytology

RS.23. The term _____ describes any restriction to the opening of the mouth caused by trauma, surgery, or radiation associated with the treatment of oral cancer.

    a. atresia

    b. cachexia

    c. steatosis

    d. trismus

RS.24. A woman who has delivered one child is referred to as a _____ .

    a. nulligravida

    b. nullipara

    c. primigravida

    d. primipara

RS.25. The term _____ means inflammation of the pancreas.

   a. pancreatalgia

   b. pancreatectomy

   c. pancreatitis

   d. pancreatotomy

RS.26. The condition in which excess cerebrospinal fluid accumulates in the ventricles of the brain is known as _____ .

   a. encephalocele

   b. hydrocephalus

   c. hydronephrosis

   d. hydroureter

RS.27. A _____ is the surgical fixation of a prolapsed vagina to a surrounding structure.

   a. colpopexy

   b. colporrhaphy

   c. cystopexy

   d. cystorrhaphy

RS.28. The combining form metr/o means _____ .

   a. breast

   b. cervix

   c. menstruation

   d. uterus

RS.29. Which statement is accurate regarding cystic fibrosis (CF)?

   a. CF is a congenital disorder in which red blood cells take on a sickle shape.

   b. CF is also known as iron overload disease.

   c. CF is a genetic disorder that affects the lungs and digestive system.

   d. CF is characterized by short-lived red blood cells.

RS.30. The condition _____ , which is thinner than average bone density, causes the patient to be at an increased risk of developing osteoporosis.

   a. osteochondroma

   b. osteopenia

   c. osteosclerosis

   d. rickets

RS.31. A/An _____ is a specialist who provides medical care to women during pregnancy, childbirth, and immediately thereafter.

   a. geriatrician

   b. gynecologist

   c. neonatologist

   d. obstetrician

RS.32. _____ is characterized by exophthalmos.

   a. Conn's syndrome

   b. Graves' disease

   c. Hashimoto's thyroiditis

   d. Huntington's disease

RS.33. The hormone _____ stimulates uterine contractions during childbirth.

   a. estrogen

   b. oxytocin

   c. progesterone

   d. testosterone

RS.34. A/An _____ is an unfavorable response due to prescribed medical treatment.

   a. idiopathic disorder

   b. nosocomial infection

   c. infectious disease

   d. iatrogenic illness

RS.35. The procedure of freeing of a kidney from adhesions is known as _____ .

   a. nephrolithiasis

   b. nephrolysis

   c. nephropyosis

   d. pyelitis

RS.36. _____ is the tissue death of an artery or arteries.

   a. Arterionecrosis

   b. Arteriostenosis

   c. Atherosclerosis

   d. Arthrosclerosis

RS.37. The _____ plane divides the body vertically into unequal left and right portions.

  a. frontal

  b. midsagittal

  c. sagittal

  d. transverse

RS.38. The term _____ means toward or nearer the midline.

  a. distal

  b. dorsal

  c. medial

  d. ventral

RS.39. A _____ was performed as a definitive test to determine if Alice Wilkinson has osteoporosis.

  a. bone marrow biopsy

  b. dual x-ray absorptiometry test

  c. MRI

  d. nuclear bone scan

RS.40. The term _____ means movement away from the midline of the body.

  a. abduction

  b. adduction

  c. extension

  d. flexion

RS.41. When he fell, Manuel tore the posterior femoral muscles in his left leg. This is known as a/an _____ injury.

  a. Achilles tendon

  b. hamstring

  c. myofascial

  d. shin splint

RS.42. Mrs. Valladares has a bacterial infection of the lining of her heart. This condition is known as bacterial _____ .

  a. endocarditis

  b. myocarditis

  c. pericarditis

  d. valvulitis

RS.43. The condition of _____ is commonly known as tooth decay.

  a. dental caries

  b. dental plaque

  c. gingivitis

  d. periodontal disease

RS.44. Henry was diagnosed as having an inflammation of the bone marrow. Which term describes this condition?

  a. encephalitis

  b. meningitis

  c. myelitis

  d. myelosis

RS.45. The term _____ describes the unnatural and irresistible urge to pull out one's own hair.

  a. acrophobia

  b. agoraphobia

  c. kleptomania

  d. trichotillomania

RS.46. The term _____ describes drooping of the upper eyelid that is usually due to paralysis.

  a. blepharoptosis

  b. dacryocystitis

  c. scleritis

  d. synechia

RS.47. The combining form _____ means old age.

  a. percuss/o

  b. presby/o

  c. prurit/o

  d. pseud/o

RS.48. Mr. Ramirez had a heart attack. His physician recorded this as _____ .

  a. angina

  b. a myocardial infarction

  c. congestive heart failure

  d. ischemic heart disease

RS.49. _____ is an abnormal increase in the number of red cells in the blood due to excess production of these cells by the bone marrow.

   a. Anemia

   b. Polycythemia

   c. Thrombocytosis

   d. Thrombocytopenia

RS.50. The common skin disorder _____ is characterized by flare-ups in which red papules covered with silvery scales occur on the elbows, knees, scalp, back, or buttocks.

   a. ichthyosis

   b. lupus erythematosus

   c. psoriasis

   d. rosacea

RS.51. _____ is a group of disorders involving the parts of the brain that control thought, memory, and language.

   a.. Alzheimer's disease

   b. Catatonic behavior

   c. Persistent vegetative state

   d. Reye's syndrome

RS.52. A/An _____ is a physician who specializes in physical medicine and rehabilitation with the focus on restoring function.

   a. exercise physiologist

   b. orthopedist

   c. physiatrist

   d. rheumatologist

RS.53. The term _____ describes a bone disorder of unknown cause that destroys normal bone structure and replaces it with fibrous tissue.

   a. costochondritis

   b. fibrous dysplasia

   c. osteomyelitis

   d. periostitis

RS.54. Slight paralysis of one side of the body is known as _____ .

   a. hemiparesis

   b. hemiplegia

   c. myoparesis

   d. quadriplegia

RS.55. The _____ are the specialized cells that play an important role in blood clotting.

   a. basophils

   b. erythrocytes

   c. leukocytes

   d. thrombocytes

RS.56. The term _____ describes blood in the urine.

   a. hemangioma

   b. hematemesis

   c. hematoma

   d. hematuria

RS.57. The _____ receives the sound vibrations and relays them to the auditory nerve fibers.

   a. cochlea

   b. eustachian tube

   c. organ of Corti

   d. semicircular canal

RS.58. The _____ patrol the body, searching for antigens that produce infections. When such a cell is found, these cells grab, swallow, and internally break apart the captured antigen.

   a. B cells

   b. dendritic cells

   c. lymphokines

   d. T cells

RS.59. The medical term for the congenital condition commonly known as clubfoot is _____ .

   a. hallux valgus

   b. rickets

   c. spasmodic torticollis

   d. talipes

RS.60. A _____ is a normal scar resulting from the healing of a wound.

   a. callus

   b. cicatrix

   c. crepitus

   d. keloid

RS.61. The _____ is commonly known as the collar bone.

    a. clavicle

    b. olecranon

    c. patella

    d. sternum

RS.62. _____ are spiral-shaped bacteria that have flexible walls and are capable of movement.

    a. Bacilli

    b. Spirochetes

    c. Staphylococcus

    d. Streptococcus

RS.63. A/An _____ is a malignant tumor usually involving the upper shaft of long bones, the pelvis, or knee.

    a. adenocarcinoma

    b. Hodgkin's lymphoma

    c. osteochondroma

    d. osteosarcoma

RS.64. Which of these diseases is transmitted to humans by mosquito or tick bites?

    a. cytomegalovirus

    b. human immunodeficiency virus

    c. rabies

    d. West Nile virus

RS.65. _____ involves compression of nerves and blood vessels due to swelling within the enclosed space created by the fascia that separates groups of muscles.

    a. Chronic fatigue syndrome

    b. Compartment syndrome

    c. Fibromyalgia syndrome

    d. Myofascial pain syndrome

RS.66. A/An _____ , also known as a *boil*, is a large, tender, swollen area caused by a staphylococcal infection around a hair follicle or sebaceous gland.

    a. abscess

    b. carbuncle

    c. furuncle

    d. pustule

RS.67. Which term refers to a class of drugs that relieves pain without affecting consciousness?

    a. analgesic

    b. barbiturate

    c. hypnotic

    d. sedative

RS.68. Fine muscle tremors, a mask-like facial expression, and a shuffling gait are all symptoms of the progressive condition known as _____ .

    a. multiple sclerosis

    b. muscular dystrophy

    c. myasthenia gravis

    d. Parkinson's disease

RS.69. _____ , formerly known as *blood poisoning*, is a systemic condition caused by the spread of microorganisms and their toxins via the circulating blood.

    a. Septicemia

    b. Botulism

    c. Tetanus

    d. Toxoplasmosis

RS.70. During her pregnancy, Ruth had a skin condition commonly known as the mask of pregnancy. The medical term for this condition is _____ .

    a. chloasma

    b. albinism

    c. melanosis

    d. vitiligo

RS.71. _____ is caused by the failure of the bones of the limbs to grow to an appropriate length.

    a. Acromegaly

    b. Gigantism

    c. Hyperpituitarism

    d. Short stature

RS.72. In a _____ fracture, one of the bones is crushed.

    a. comminuted

    b. compound

    c. compression

    d. spiral

RS.73. The combining form _____ means vertebra or vertebral column.

    a. synovi/o

    b. spondyl/o

    c. scoli/o

    d. splen/o

RS.74. Which heart chamber receives oxygen-poor blood from all tissues, except the lungs?

    a. left atrium

    b. left ventricle

    c. right atrium

    d. right ventricle

RS.75. Which substance is commonly known as good cholesterol?

    a. high-density lipoprotein cholesterol

    b. homocysteine

    c. low-density lipoprotein cholesterol

    d. triglycerides

RS.76. Which symbol means less than?

    a. $>$

    b. $\geq$

    c. $<$

    d. $\leq$

RS.77. When medication is placed under the tongue and allowed to dissolve slowly, this is known as _____ administration.

    a. oral

    b. parenteral

    c. sublingual

    d. topical

RS.78. A sonogram is the image created by _____ .

    a. computerized tomography

    b. fluoroscopy

    c. magnetic resonance imaging (MRI)

    d. ultrasonography

RS.79. Which combining form means red?

    a. melan/o

    b. leuk/o

    c. erythr/o

    d. cyan/o

RS.80. The surgical puncture of the eardrum with a needle to remove fluid or pus from an infected middle ear is known as _____ .

    a. abdominocentesis

    b. arthrocentesis

    c. thoracentesis

    d. tympanocentesis

RS.81. The term _____ describes inflammation of the gallbladder.

    a. cholecystectomy

    b. cholecystitis

    c. cholecystotomy

    d. cholelithiasis

RS.82. The term _____ means vomiting.

    a. emesis

    b. epistaxis

    c. reflux

    d. singultus

RS.83. The bluish discoloration of the skin caused by a lack of adequate oxygen is known as _____ .

    a. cyanosis

    b. erythema

    c. jaundice

    d. pallor

RS.84. _____ is a disorder of the adrenal glands due to excessive production of aldosterone.

    a. Conn's syndrome

    b. Crohn's disease

    c. Cushing's syndrome

    d. Raynaud's phenomenon

RS.85. A/An _____ is any substance that the body regards as being foreign.

    a. allergen

    b. antibody

    c. antigen

    d. immunoglobulin

RS.86. Which condition has purple discolorations on the skin due to bleeding underneath the skin?

    a. dermatosis

    b. pruritus

    c. purpura

    d. suppuration

RS.87. _____ is an excessive fear of spiders.

    a. Acrophobia

    b. Agoraphobia

    c. Arachnophobia

    d. Claustrophobia

RS.88. A band of fibrous tissue that holds structures together abnormally is a/an _____ .

    a. adhesion

    b. ankylosis

    c. contracture

    d. ligation

RS.89. Which procedure is performed to treat spider veins?

    a. blepharoplasty

    b. Botox

    c. liposuction

    d. sclerotherapy

RS.90. The instrument used to view the interior of the ear canal is known as a/an _____ .

    a. anoscope

    b. ophthalmoscope

    c. otoscope

    d. speculum

RS.91. Which condition is breast cancer at its earliest stage before the cancer has broken through the wall of the milk duct?

    a. ductal carcinoma in situ

    b. infiltrating lobular carcinoma

    c. inflammatory breast cancer

    d. invasive lobular carcinoma

RS.92. Enlarged and swollen veins at the lower end of the esophagus are known as _____ .

    a. esophageal aneurisms

    b. esophageal varices

    c. hemorrhoids

    d. varicose veins

RS.93. _____ is a progressive autoimmune disorder characterized by scattered patches of demyelination of nerve fibers of the brain and spinal cord.

    a. Lupus erythematosus

    b. Multiple sclerosis

    c. Muscular dystrophy

    d. Spina bifida

RS.94. The abdominal region located below the stomach is known as the _____ region.

    a. epigastric

    b. hypogastric

    c. left hypochondriac

    d. umbilical

RS.95. Which of these sexually transmitted disease is a bacterial infection?

    a. acquired immunodeficiency syndrome

    b. gonorrhea

    c. genital herpes

    d. trichomoniasis

RS.96. Narrowing of the opening of the foreskin so that it cannot be retracted to expose the glans penis is known as _____ .

    a. balanitis

    b. Peyronie's disease

    c. phimosis

    d. priapism

RS.97. A/An _____ is an exfoliative screening biopsy for the detection and diagnosis of conditions of the cervix and surrounding tissues.

    a. endometrial biopsy

    b. lymph node dissection

    c. Papanicolaou test

    d. sentinel node biopsy

RS.98. In the field of assisted fertilization, the abbreviation AMA stands for _____ .

    a. advanced maternal age

    b. against medical advice

    c. American Medical Association

    d. American Mother's Association

RS.99. The term _____ describes turning the palm upward or forward.

    a. circumduction

    b. pronation

    c. rotation

    d. supination

RS.100. The term _____ describes the inflammation of a vein.

    a. angiitis

    b. arteritis

    c. phlebitis

    d. phlebostenosis

Simulated Final Test

FT.1. The term _____ describes a torn or ragged wound.

    a. fissure

    b. fistula

    c. laceration

    d. lesion

FT.2. The bone and soft tissues that surround and support the teeth are known as the _____ .

    a. dentition

    b. rugae

    c. gingiva

    d. periodontium

FT.3. A chronic condition in which the heart is unable to pump out all of the blood that it receives is known as _____ .

    a. atrial fibrillation

    b. congestive heart failure

    c. tachycardia

    d. ventricular fibrillation

FT.4. Inflammation of the connective tissues that encloses the spinal cord and brain is known as _____ .

    a. encephalitis

    b. encephalopathy

    c. meningitis

    d. myelopathy

FT.5. _____ is the partial or complete blockage of the small and/or large intestine that is caused by the cessation of intestinal peristalsis.

    a. Crohn's disease

    b. Ileus

    c. Intussusception

    d. Intestinal obstruction

FT.6. The term _____ describes a condition in which the eye does not focus properly because of uneven curvatures of the cornea.

    a. ametropia

    b. astigmatism

    c. ectropion

    d. entropion

FT.7. Which term means abnormal softening of the kidney?

    a. nephromalacia

    b. nephrosclerosis

    c. neuromalacia

    d. neurosclerosis

FT.8. The term _____ describes persistent severe burning pain that usually follows an injury to a sensory nerve.

    a. causalgia

    b. hyperesthesia

    c. paresthesia

    d. peripheral neuropathy

FT.9. A/An _____ is performed to reduce the risk of a stroke caused by a disruption of the blood flow to the brain.

    a. aneurysmectomy

    b. arteriectomy

    c. carotid endarterectomy

    d. coronary artery bypass graft

FT.10. The term _____ means bleeding from the ear.

    a. barotrauma

    b. otomycosis

    c. otopyorrhea

    d. otorrhagia

FT.11. The medical term meaning itching is _____ .

    a. perfusion

    b. pruritus

    c. purpura

    d. suppuration

FT.12. _____ is a condition characterized by episodes of severe chest pain due to inadequate blood flow to the myocardium.

    a. Angina

    b. Claudication

    c. Cyanosis

    d. Myocardial infarction

FT.13. The greenish material that forms the first stools of a newborn is known as _____ .

    a. colostrum

    b. lochia

    c. meconium

    d. vernix

FT.14. A/An _____ is the result of medical treatment that yields the exact opposite of normally-expected results.

    a. drug interaction

    b. paradoxical reaction

    c. placebo

    d. potentiation

FT.15. A _____ is a prediction of the probable course and outcome of a disease or disorder.

    a. differential diagnosis

    b. diagnosis

    c. prognosis

    d. syndrome

FT.16. _____ is a yellow discoloration of the skin, mucous membranes, and the eyes.

    a. Vitiligo

    b. Jaundice

    c. Erythema

    d. Albinism

FT.17. A/An _____ occurs at the lower end of the radius when a person tries to break a fall by landing on his or her hands.

    a. Colles' fracture

    b. comminuted fracture

    c. osteoporotic hip fracture

    d. spiral fracture

FT.18. The term _____ describes excessive urination during the night.

    a. nocturia

    b. polydipsia

    c. polyuria

    d. urinary retention

FT.19. A closed sac associated with a sebaceous gland that contains yellow, fatty material is known as a _____ .

    a. comedo

    b. sebaceous cyst

    c. seborrheic dermatitis

    d. seborrheic keratosis

FT.20. The term _____ describes the condition commonly known as swollen glands.

    a. adenoiditis

    b. angiitis

    c. lymphadenitis

    d. lymphangioma

FT.21. A/An _____ is a sudden, violent, involuntary contraction of one or more muscles.

    a. adhesion

    b. contracture

    c. spasm

    d. sprain

FT.22. _____ is the respiratory disease commonly known as whooping cough.

    a. Coup

    b. Diphtheria

    c. Emphysema

    d. Pertussis

FT.23. The bone disorder of unknown cause that destroys normal bone structure and replaces it with scar-like tissue is known as _____ .

    a. ankylosing spondylitis

    b. fibrous dysplasia

    c. Paget's disease

    d. Wilms tumor

FT.24. _____ is an abnormal lateral curvature of the spine.

    a. Kyphosis

    b. Lordosis

    c. Lumbago

    d. Scoliosis

FT.25. The surgical creation of an artificial excretory opening between the ileum and the outside of the abdominal wall is a/an _____ .

    a. colostomy

    b. enteropexy

    c. gastroptosis

    d. ileostomy

FT.26. Which examination technique is the visualization of body parts in motion by projecting x-ray images on a luminous fluorescent screen?

    a. computed tomography

    b. fluoroscopy

    c. magnetic resonance imaging

    d. radiography

FT.27. As the condition known as _____ progresses, the chest sometimes assumes an enlarged barrel shape.

    a. asthma

    b. diphtheria

    c. emphysema

    d. epistaxis

FT.28. The term _____ means to stop or control bleeding.

    a. hemorrhage

    b. hemostasis

    c. homeostasis

    d. thrombocytopenia

FT.29. An accumulation of pus in the fallopian tube is known as _____ .

    a. leukorrhea

    b. otopyorrhea

    c. pyosalpinx

    d. salpingitis

FT.30. A _____ is the bruising of brain tissue as a result of a head injury.

    a. cerebral contusion

    b. concussion

    c. hydrocele

    d. meningocele

FT.31. The term _____ means vomiting blood.

    a. epistaxis

    b. hemarthrosis

    c. hematemesis

    d. hyperemesis

FT.32. _____ is a diagnostic procedure designed to determine the density of a body part by the sound produced by tapping the surface with the fingers.

    a. Auscultation

    b. Palpation

    c. Percussion

    d. Range of motion

FT.33. Abnormally rapid, deep breathing resulting in decreased levels of carbon dioxide at the cellular level is known as _____ .

    a. apnea

    b. dyspnea

    c. hyperventilation

    d. hypoventilation

FT.34. The term _____ describes difficult or painful urination.

    a. dyspepsia

    b. dysphagia

    c. dystrophy

    d. dysuria

FT.35. A _____ is a false personal belief that is maintained despite obvious proof to the contrary.

    a. delusion

    b. dementia

    c. mania

    d. phobia

FT.36. In _____ , the normal rhythmic contractions of the atria are replaced by rapid irregular twitching of the muscular wall of the heart.

    a. atrial fibrillation

    b. bradycardia

    c. tachycardia

    d. ventricular fibrillation

FT.37. The eye condition known as _____ is characterized by increased intraocular pressure.

   a. cataracts

   b. glaucoma

   c. macular degeneration

   d. monochromatism

FT.38. _____ is the presence of blood in the seminal fluid.

   a. Azoospermia

   b. Hematuria

   c. Hemospermia

   d. Prostatorrhea

FT.39. The condition of common changes in the eyes that occur with aging is known as _____ .

   a. hyperopia

   b. presbycusis

   c. presbyopia

   d. strabismus

FT.40. Which body cavity protects the brain?

   a. anterior

   b. cranial

   c. caudal

   d. ventral

FT.41. A hernia of the bladder through the vaginal wall is known as a _____ .

   a. cystocele

   b. cystopexy

   c. vaginocele

   d. vesicovaginal fistula

FT.42. Which condition of a young child is characterized by the inability to develop normal social relationships?

   a. autism

   b. attention deficit disorder

   c. dyslexia

   d. mental retardation

FT.43. A ringing, buzzing, or roaring sound in one or both ears is known as _____ .

   a. labyrinthitis

   b. syncope

   c. tinnitus

   d. vertigo

FT.44. A/An _____ is an outbreak of a disease occurring over a large geographic area that is possibly worldwide.

   a. endemic

   b. epidemic

   c. pandemic

   d. syndrome

FT.45. _____ is an abnormal accumulation of serous fluid in the peritoneal cavity.

   a. Ascites

   b. Aerophagia

   c. Melena

   d. Steatosis

FT.46. A _____ is a small, flat, discolored lesion such as a freckle.

   a. macule

   b. papule

   c. plaque

   d. vesicle

FT.47. The Western blot test is used to _____ .

   a. confirm an HIV infection

   b. detect hepatitis C

   c. diagnose Kaposi's sarcoma

   d. test for tuberculosis

FT.48. The term _____ describes excessive uterine bleeding at both the usual time of menstrual periods and at other irregular intervals.

   a. dysmenorrhea

   b. hypermenorrhea

   c. menometrorrhagia

   d. oligomenorrhea

FT.49. _____ is a form of sexual dysfunction in which the penis is bent or curved during erection.

   a. Anorchism

   b. Peyronie's disease

   c. Phimosis

   d. Priapism

FT.50. A/An _____ is an abnormal harsh or musical sound heard during of auscultation of an artery.

a. auscultation

b. bruit

c. rhonchus

d. stridor

FT.51. The condition commonly known as wear-and-tear arthritis is _____ .

a. gouty arthritis

b. osteoarthritis

c. rheumatoid arthritis

d. spondylosis

FT.52. The term _____ means to free a tendon from adhesions.

a. tenodesis

b. tenolysis

c. tenorrhaphy

d. tenoplasty

FT.53. The malignant condition known as _____ is distinguished by the presence of Reed-Sternberg cells.

a. Hodgkin's lymphoma

b. leukemia

c. non-Hodgkin's lymphoma

d. osteosarcoma

FT.54. The progressive, degenerative disease characterized by disturbance of structure and function of the liver is _____ .

a. cirrhosis

b. hepatitis

c. hepatomegaly

d. jaundice

FT.55. _____ removes waste products directly from the bloodstream of patients whose kidneys no longer function.

a. Diuresis

b. Epispadias

c. Hemodialysis

d. Peritoneal dialysis

FT.56. The medical term for the condition commonly known as fainting is _____ .

a. comatose

b. singultus

c. stupor

d. syncope

FT.57. _____ is a condition in which the oxygen supply is insufficient to a part of the body because of restricted blood flow.

a. Angina

b. Infarction

c. Ischemia

d. Perfusion

FT.58. A collection of blood in the pleural cavity is known as a _____ .

a. hemophilia

b. hemoptysis

c. hemostasis

d. hemothorax

FT.59. The return of swallowed food into the mouth is known as _____ .

a. dysphagia

b. emesis

c. pyrosis

d. regurgitation

FT.60. An inflammation of the lacrimal gland that can be a bacterial, viral, or fungal infection is known as _____ .

a. anisocoria

b. dacryoadenitis

c. exophthalmos

d. hordeolum

FT.61. The yellow discoloration of the skin, mucous membranes, and white of the eyes caused by excessive amounts of bilirubin in the blood, is known as _____ .

a. albinism

b. cyanosis

c. jaundice

d. melanosis

FT.62. The term _____ means excessive urination.

   a. enuresis

   b. oliguria

   c. overactive bladder

   d. polyuria

FT.63. The surgical removal of the gallbladder is known as a _____ .

   a. cholecystectomy

   b. cholecystostomy

   c. cholecystotomy

   d. choledocholithotomy

FT.64. An elevated _____ indicates the presence of inflammation in the body.

   a. complete blood cell count

   b. erythrocyte sedimentation rate

   c. platelet count

   d. total hemoglobin test

FT.65. A/An _____ is a groove or crack-like sore or break in the skin.

   a. abrasion

   b. fissure

   c. laceration

   d. ulcer

FT.66. A/An _____ injection is made into the fatty layer just below the skin.

   a. intradermal

   b. intramuscular

   c. intravenous

   d. subcutaneous

FT.67. The _____ has roles in both the immune and endocrine systems.

   a. pancreas

   b. pituitary

   c. spleen

   d. thymus

FT.68. The medical term _____ describes an inflammation of the brain.

   a. encephalitis

   b. mastitis

   c. meningitis

   d. myelitis

FT.69. The hormone secreted by fat cells is known as _____ .

   a. interstitial cell-stimulating hormone

   b. growth hormone

   c. leptin

   d. neurohormone

FT.70. When the body has too much thyroid hormone due to taking too much thyroid hormone medication, the condition known as _____ develops.

   a. factitious hyperthyroidism

   b. goiter

   c. myxedema

   d. thyroid storm

FT.71. A/An _____ is acquired in a hospital or clinic setting.

   a. functional disorder

   b. iatrogenic illness

   c. idiopathic disorder

   d. nosocomial infection

FT.72. _____ is breast cancer at its earliest stage before the cancer has broken through the wall of the milk duct.

   a. Ductal carcinoma in situ

   b. Infiltrating ductal carcinoma

   c. Infiltrating lobular carcinoma

   d. Inflammatory breast cancer

FT.73. The term _____ describes an eye disorder that can develop as a complication of diabetes.

   a. diabetic neuropathy

   b. diabetic retinopathy

   c. papilledema

   d. retinal detachment

FT.74. The physical wasting with the loss of weight and muscle mass due to diseases such as advanced cancer is known as _____ .

   a. cachexia

   b. anorexia nervosa

   c. bulimia nervosa

   d. malnutrition

FT.75. The term _____ means difficulty in swallowing.

    a. aerophagia

    b. dyspepsia

    c. dysphagia

    d. eructation

FT.76. A/An _____ occurs when a blood vessel in the brain leaks or ruptures.

    a. cerebral hematoma

    b. embolism

    c. hemorrhagic stroke

    d. ischemic stroke

FT.77. The hormonal disorder known as _____ results from the pituitary gland producing too much growth hormone in adults.

    a. acromegaly

    b. cretinism

    c. gigantism

    d. pituitarism

FT.78. The term _____ describes the condition commonly known an ingrown toenail.

    a. cryptorchidism

    b. onychocryptosis

    c. onychomycosis

    d. priapism

FT.79. An _____ is the instrument used to examine the interior of the eye.

    a. ophtalmoscope

    b. ophthalmoscope

    c. opthalmoscope

    d. opthlmoscope

FT.80. A/An _____ is a protrusion of part of the stomach through the esophageal sphincter in the diaphragm.

    a. esophageal hernia

    b. esophageal varices

    c. hiatal hernia

    d. hiatal varices

FT.81. An _____ is a surgical incision made to enlarge the vaginal orifice to facilitate childbirth.

    a. episiorrhaphy

    b. episiotomy

    c. epispadias

    d. epistaxis

FT.82. Severe itching of the external female genitalia is known as _____ .

    a. colpitis

    b. leukorrhea

    c. oruritus vulvae

    d. vaginal candidiasis

FT.83. _____ is a urinary problem caused by interference with the normal nerve pathways associated with urination.

    a. Neurogenic bladder

    b. Overactive bladder

    c. Polyuria

    d. Trigonitis

FT.84. A/An _____ is used to enlarge the opening of a canal or body cavity to make it possible to inspect its interior.

    a. endoscope

    b. speculum

    c. sphygmomanometer

    d. stethoscope

FT.85. A _____ , also known as *scab*, is a collection of dried serum and cellular debris.

    a. crust

    b. nodule

    c. plaque

    d. scale

FT.86. A _____ is a type of cancer that occurs in blood-making cells found in the red bone marrow.

    a. carcinoma

    b. myeloma

    c. osteochondroma

    d. sarcoma

FT.87. _____ can occur when a foreign substance, such as vomit, is inhaled into the lungs.

    a. Aspiration pneumonia

    b. Bacterial pneumonia

    c. Mycoplasma pneumonia

    d. Pneumocystis carinii pneumonia

FT.88. The condition known as _____ , is ankylosis of the bones of the middle ear that causes a conductive hearing loss.

   a. labyrinthitis

   b. mastoiditis

   c. osteosclerosis

   d. otosclerosis

FT.89. The procedure known as _____ , is the surgical fusion of two bones to stiffen a joint.

   a. arthrodesis

   b. arthrolysis

   c. synovectomy

   d. tenodesis

FT.90. The suffix _____ means rupture.

   a. -rrhage

   b. -rrhaphy

   c. -rrhea

   d. -rrhexis

FT.91. An abnormal fear of being in narrow or enclosed spaces is known as _____ .

   a. acrophobia

   b. agoraphobia

   c. arachnophobia

   d. claustrophobia

FT.92. _____ is the distortion, or impairment, of voluntary movement such as in a tic or spasm.

   a. Bradykinesia

   b. Dyskinesia

   c. Hyperkinesia

   d. Myoclonus

FT.93. Which structure secretes bile?

   a. gallbladder

   b. liver

   c. pancreas

   d. spleen

FT.94. _____ is the process of recording electrical brain wave activity.

   a. Echoencephalograph

   b. Electroencephalography

   c. Electromyography

   d. Electroneuromyography

FT.95. The suffix _____ means surgical fixation.

   a. - rrhagia

   b. -rrhaphy

   c. - rrhea

   d. -rrhexis

FT.96. The eye condition that causes the loss of central vision, but not total blindness, is known as _____ .

   a. cataracts

   b. glaucoma

   c. macular degeneration

   d. presbyopia

FT.97. A/An _____ is performed to remove excess skin for the elimination of wrinkles.

   a. ablation

   b. blepharoplasty

   c. rhytidectomy

   d. sclerotherapy

FT.98. The condition known as _____ describes total paralysis affecting only one side of the body.

   a. hemiparesis

   b. hemiplegia

   c. paraplegia

   d. quadriplegia

FT.99. _____ is a new cancer site that results from the spreading process.

   a. In situ

   b. Metabolism

   c. Metastasis

   d. Metastasize

FT.100. Which of these hormone is produced by the pituitary gland?

   a. adrenocorticotropic hormone

   b. calcitonin

   c. cortisol

   d. epinephrine

Notes

Notes

Notes

Notes

Notes

Notes

Notes

Notes

Notes

Notes

Notes

Notes

Notes

Notes

Notes

Notes

Flash Cards

INSTRUCTIONS

- Carefully remove the flash card pages from the workbook and separate them to create 160 flash cards.

- There are three types of cards: **prefixes** (such as a- and hyper-), **suffixes** (such as -graphy and -rrhagia), and **word roots/combining forms** (such as gastr/o and arthr/o). For the prefixes and suffixes, the type of word part is listed on the front of each card and the definition is on the back.

- The word root/combining form cards are arranged by body systems. This allows you to sort out the cards you want to study based on where you are in the book. Use the "general" cards as they apply throughout your course.

- Use the flash cards to memorize word parts, to test yourself, and to serve as a periodic review.

- By putting cards together, you can create terms just as you did in the challenge word building exercises.

WORD PART GAMES

Here are games you can play with one or more partners to help you learn word parts using your flash cards.

The Review Game

Word Parts Up: Shuffle the deck of flash cards. Put the pile, *word parts up*, in the center of the desk. Take turns choosing a card from anywhere in the deck and giving the definition of the word part shown. If you get it right, you get to keep it. If you miss, it goes into the discard pile. When the draw pile is gone, whoever has the largest pile wins.

Definitions Up: Shuffle the deck of flash cards and place them with the *definition side up*. Play the review game the same way.

The Create-a-Word Game

Shuffle the deck and deal each person 14 cards, *word parts up*. Place the remaining draw pile in the center of the desk, *word parts down*.

Each player should try to create as many legitimate medical words as possible using the cards he or she has been dealt, then take turns discarding one card (word part up, in the discard pile) and taking one. When it is your turn to discard a card, you may choose either the card the previous player discarded, or a "mystery card" from the draw pile. Continue working on words until all the cards in the draw pile have been taken.

To score, each player must define every word created correctly. If the definition is correct, the player receives one point for each card used. If it is incorrect, two points are deducted for each card in that word. Cards left unused each count as one point off. Whoever has the highest number of points wins. Note: Use your medical dictionary if there is any doubt that a word is legitimate!

A-, AN-

ANTE-

ANTI-

BRADY-

DYS-

END-, ENDO-

HEMI-

HYPER-

HYPO-

INTER-

within, in, inside	without, away from, negative, not
half	before, toward
excessive, increased	against, counter
deficient, decreased	slow
between, among	bad, difficult, painful

prefix

INTRA-

prefix

POST-

prefix

NEO-

prefix

PRE-

prefix

PER-

prefix

SUB-

prefix

PERI-

prefix

SUPER-, SUPRA-

prefix

POLY-

prefix

TACHY-

after	within, inside
before	new, strange
below	excessive, through
above, excessive	surrounding, around
fast, rapid	many

-AC, -AL

-CYTE

-ALGIA

-DESIS

-ARY

-ECTOMY

-CELE

-ECTASIS

-CENTESIS

-EMIA

cell	pertaining to, relating to
surgical fixation of bone or joint, to bind, tie together	pain, suffering
surgical removal	pertaining to
stretching, enlargement	hernia, tumor, swelling
blood, blood condition	surgical puncture to remove fluid

suffix

-ESTHESIA

suffix

-ITIS

suffix

-GRAM, -GRAPH

suffix

-LYSIS

suffix

-GRAPHY

suffix

-MALACIA

suffix

-IA

suffix

-MEGALY

suffix

-IC

suffix

-NECROSIS

inflammation	sensation, feeling
breakdown, separation, setting free, destruction, loosening	a picture or record
abnormal softening	the process of recording a picture or record
enlargement	state or condition
tissue death	pertaining to

-OLOGIST

-OTOMY

-OLOGY

-PATHY

-OMA

-PAUSE

-OSIS

-PEXY

-OSTOMY

-PLASTY

surgical incision	specialist
disease, suffering, feeling, emotion	the science or study of
stopping	tumor
surgical fixation, to put in place	abnormal condition
surgical repair	surgical creation of an opening

-PLEGIA

-RRHEA

-PNEA

-RRHEXIS

-PTOSIS

-SCLEROSIS

**-RRHAGIA,
-RRHAGE**

-SCOPE

-RRHAPHY

-SCOPY

abnormal flow or discharge	paralysis
rupture	breathing
abnormal hardening	prolapse, drooping forward
instrument for visual examination	bleeding, abnormal excessive fluid discharge
to see, visual examination	to suture

-STENOSIS

ARTER/O, ARTERI/O

-TRIPSY

ATHER/O

-URIA

CARD/O, CARDI/O

ANGI/O

HEM/O, HEMAT/O

AORT/O

PHLEB/O

artery	abnormal narrowing
plaque, fatty substance	to crush
heart	urination, urine
blood, pertaining to the blood	pertaining to blood or lymph vessels
vein	aorta

Cardiovascular System	Digestive System
THROMB/O	**COL/O, COLON/O**
Cardiovascular System	Digestive System
VEN/O	**DUODEN/I, DUODEN/O**
Diagnostic Procedures	Digestive System
ECH/O	**ENTER/O**
Diagnostic Procedures	Digestive System
RADI/O	**ESOPHAG/O**
Digestive System	Digestive System
CHOLECYST/O	**GASTR/O**

colon, large intestine	clot
duodenum	vein
small intestine	sound
esophagus	radiation, x-rays
stomach	gallbladder

HEPAT/O

THYR/O, THYROID/O

SIGMOID/O

ADIP/O

ADREN/O, ADRENAL/O

ALBIN/O

GONAD/O

CEPHAL/O

PANCREAT/O

CERVIC/O

thyroid gland

liver

fat

sigmoid colon

white

adrenal glands

head

sex gland

neck, cervix
(neck of uterus)

pancreas

General

CORON/O

General

CYAN/O

General

CYT/O

General

ERYTHR/O

General

HIST/O

General

LAPAR/O

General

LEUK/O

General

LIP/O

General

MELAN/O

General

MYC/O

abdomen, abdominal wall	coronary, crown
white	blue
fat, lipid	cell
black, dark	red
fungus	tissue

General	Immune System
PATH/O	**ONC/O**

General	Integumentary System
PY/O	**CUTANE/O**

General	Integumentary System
PYR/O	**DERM/O, DERMAT/O**

General	Integumentary System
SARC/O	**HIDR/O**

Immune System	Integumentary System
CARCIN/O	**SEB/O**

tumor	disease, suffering, feeling, emotion
skin	pus
skin	fever, fire
sweat	flesh (connective tissue)
sebum	cancerous

Integumentary System	Muscular System
UNGU/O	**MY/O**
Integumentary System	Muscular System
XER/O	**TEN/O, TEND/O, TENDIN/O**
Lymphatic System	Nervous System
ADEN/O	**ENCEPHAL/O**
Lymphatic System	Nervous System
SPLEN/O	**MENING/O**
Muscular System	Nervous System
FASCI/O	**NEUR/I, NEUR/O**

muscle	nail
tendon, stretch out, extend, strain	dry
brain	gland
meninges	spleen
nerve, nerve tissue	fascia, fibrous band

COLP/O

OOPHOR/O, OVARI/O

HYSTER/O

ORCH/O, ORCHI/O, ORCHID/O

MEN/O

SALPING/O

METR/O, METRI/O

UTER/O

OO/O, OV/I, OV/O

VAGIN/O

ovary

vagina

testicles, testis, testes

uterus

uterine (fallopian) tube,
auditory (eustachian) tube

menstruation, menses

uterus

uterus

vagina

egg

Respiratory System

Respiratory System

**BRONCH/O,
BRONCHI/O**

**PULM/O,
PULMON/O**

Respiratory System

Respiratory System

LARYNG/O

TRACHE/O

Respiratory System

Skeletal System

PHARYNG/O

ANKLY/O

Respiratory System

Skeletal System

PLEUR/O

ARTHR/O

Respiratory System

Skeletal System

**PNEUM/O,
PNEUMON/O**

CHONDR/O

lung	bronchial tube, bronchus
trachea, windpipe	larynx, voice box
crooked, bent, stiff	throat, pharynx
joint	pleura, side of the body
cartilage	lung, air

Skeletal System	Skeletal & Respiratory Systems
COST/O	**THORAC/O**

Skeletal System	Special Senses & Integumentary System
CRANI/O	**KERAT/O**

Skeletal System & Nervous System	Special Senses
MYEL/O	**MYRING/O**

Skeletal System	Special Senses
OSS/E, OSS/I, OST/O, OSTE/O	**OPTIC/O, OPT/O**

Skeletal System	Special Senses
SPONDYL/O	**OT/O**

chest

rib

horny, hard, cornea

skull

tympanic membrane,
eardrum

spinal cord,
bone marrow

eye, vision

bone

ear, hearing

vertebrae, vertebral
column, back bone

Special Senses	Urinary System
RETIN/O	**NEPHR/O**
Special Senses & Integumentary System	Urinary System
SCLER/O	**PYEL/O**
Special Senses	Urinary System
TYMPAN/O	**REN/O**
Urinary System	Urinary System
CYST/O	**URETER/O**
Urinary System & Digestive System	Urinary System
LITH/O	**URETHR/O**

kidney	retina
renal pelvis, bowl of kidney	sclera, white of eye, hard
kidney	tympanic membrane, eardrum
ureter	urinary bladder, cyst, sac of fluid
urethra	stone, calculus